Crohn's Disease

AND

Ulcerative Colitis

EVERYTHING YOU NEED TO KNOW
THE COMPLETE PRACTICAL GUIDE

THIRD EDITION

Fred Saibil, M.D.

FIREFLY BOOKS

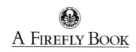

A FIREFLY BOOK

Published by Firefly Books Ltd. 2011

First printing

Publisher Cataloging-in-Publication Data (U.S.)

Saibil, Fred.
Crohn's disease and ulcerative colitis : everything you need to know / Fred Saibil, M.D. — 3rd ed.
[248] p. : cm.
Includes index.

ISBN-13: 978-1-55407-645-1 (pbk.)

1. Crohn's disease. 2. Ulcerative colitis. I. Title.
616.344 dc22   RC862.E52S353 2011

Library and Archives Canada Cataloguing in Publication

Saibil, Fredric G., 1942-
Crohn's disease and ulcerative colitis : everything you need to know / Fred Saibil.
— 3rd ed.
Includes index.

ISBN-13: 978-1-55407-645-1

1. Crohn's disease—Popular works. 2. Ulcerative colitis—Popular works. I. Title.
RC862.I53S25 2011   616.3'44
C2011-902323-7

Published in the United States by
Firefly Books (U.S.) Inc.
P.O. Box 1338, Ellicott Station
Buffalo, New York 14205

Published in Canada by
Firefly Books Ltd.
66 Leek Crescent
Richmond Hill, Ontario L4B 1H1

Printed in Canada

The publisher gratefully acknowledges the financial support for our publishing program by the Government of Canada through the Canada Book Fund as administered by the Department of Canadian Heritage.

Contents

DISCLAIMER

It is important that you read all following terms and conditions carefully. **All medical content is intended for residents of Canada only.** The subject matter provided in this book is for informational purposes only and is not professional medical advice, diagnosis, treatment or care, nor is it intended to a be a substitute therefor. The content of this book does not establish a doctor-patient relationship. You should always seek the advice of your physicians or other members of your treatment team concerning any questions you may have regarding any content obtained from this book. This should be done prior to following any of the management suggestions. Never disregard professional medical advice or delay in seeking it because of something you have read in this book. Always consult with your physician or other members of your treatment team before embarking on a new treatment or diet. The content of this book is not exhaustive and does not cover all diseases, ailments, physical conditions or their treatment.

Do not use this book for medical emergencies. If you have a medical emergency, call a physician, a qualified healthcare provider, or 911 (or the applicable local emergency number) immediately. In the event of an emergency, under no circumstances should you attempt self-treatment or treatment of someone else based on anything you have seen or read in this book.

The book and its content are provided "AS IS." While the author endeavors to provide content that is correct, accurate, current and timely, the author makes no representations, warranties, conditions, or covenants, express or implied, that the content will be accurate, complete, current, reliable, or error-free. The reader acknowledges and agrees use of this book and its content is entirely at your own risk and liability.

In no event shall the author be liable for damages of any kind, including, without limitation, any direct, special, indirect, punitive, incidental or consequential damages including, without limitation, any loss or damages in the nature of, or relating to, lost business, medical injury, personal injury, wrongful death, emotional harm, improper diagnosis, inaccurate information, improper treatment or any other loss incurred in connection with your use, misuse or reliance upon the book or its content. The foregoing limitation shall apply even if the author knew or ought to have known of the possibility of such damages. The author also expressly disclaims any and all liability for the acts, omissions or conduct of any third party user-advertiser. Under no circumstances shall the author be liable for any injury, loss, damage (including direct, special, indirect, punitive, incidental or consequential damages), or expense arising in any manner whatsoever from the acts, omissions or conduct of any third party. The foregoing limitation shall apply even if the author knew of or ought to have known of the possibility of such damages. Unless specifically stated, the author does not recommend or endorse any specific brand of products or services that appears or that may be advertised in this book.

The book contains links to third-party websites. These links are provided solely as a convenience to the reader and not as an endorsement by the author of any third-party website or the content thereof.

To my friend Dr. David Sachar, a consummate scholar, a compassionate and knowledgeable physician, a world-renowned expert in inflammatory bowel disease and my foremost mentor.

Dr. Sachar presented the following quotation at an international meeting of IBD experts, and I can think of no better way to describe the needs of people with inflammatory bowel disease and various other chronic diseases:

> Time personally spent with the patient is the most essential ingredient of excellence in clinical practice. There are simply no short cuts and no substitutions . . . There must be time to assess the patient's intellectual and psychological elements; time to meticulously gather each piece of clinical evidence from the history and physical examination; time to analyze these data and add them to other helpful information from special studies and consultations; time to evolve a plan of management when diagnostic conclusions have been reached. And, above all, there must be time for the patient to communicate himself to you, and you to him. Without adequate time, you cannot possibly give sufficiently of yourself to your patients. Time is what they expect and what they need. (P.A. Tumulty, "The Art of Healing," *Johns Hopkins Medical Journal* 143 [1978]: 140–43.)

Introduction

The term "inflammatory bowel disease" (IBD) refers mainly to Crohn's disease and ulcerative colitis, two closely related conditions that cause persistent or recurring inflammation of one or more parts of the intestine. Whereas Crohn's disease can affect any part of the gastrointestinal system, from the mouth to the anus, ulcerative colitis occurs only in the colon (large intestine, large bowel). Some people include three other conditions under the IBD heading: microscopic colitis (including lymphocytic colitis and collagenous colitis), segmental colitis associated with diverticulosis (SCAD) and Behçet's disease. But, by convention, when someone says "IBD," they are referring to Crohn's disease and ulcerative colitis.

Descriptions compatible with both ulcerative colitis and Crohn's disease first appeared several centuries ago, but they did not attract general medical interest until the last half of the 19th century. Sir Samuel Wilks, a distinguished British physician, first used the term "ulcerative colitis" in a case report published in 1859 in London, England. In 1913, a Scottish surgeon named Dalziel wrote an article in a British journal describing a group of nine patients with what was probably Crohn's disease. But it wasn't until 1932, when a more widely publicized report reemphasizing Dalziel's findings was published in the United States by Dr. Burrill Crohn and his colleagues at the Mount Sinai Medical Center in New York City, that the disease came to be known as Crohn's disease.

The causes of Crohn's disease and ulcerative colitis are unknown. For years these conditions were thought to be due to stress, but we now know this is not the case. Current thought is that people are born with an inherited tendency to get IBD, and then one or more things in the environment come along and trigger the onset of the disease. IBD can start at any age but usually begins in the late teens or early adulthood. Both Crohn's disease and ulcerative colitis are sometimes associated with various medical problems outside of the intestine, including arthritis, skin conditions, kidney stones, cancer and gallstones. There is no known cure for Crohn's disease; ulcerative colitis can be cured, but only by surgical removal of the whole colon, including the rectum.

Managing a chronic disease requires a team effort, the team consisting of the patient (and possibly the patient's family), the doctor (and possibly additional doctors) and, sometimes, other health-care professionals. If patients are taught which problems they can treat (or at least start to treat) themselves, and which ones should be promptly reported, they achieve a greater degree of independence. For many patients, this means being able to go about their daily lives without worry.

This book, which is aimed primarily at patients and their families, provides a comprehensive review of IBD and many principles of self-management. Every effort has been made to avoid complex medical terminology. When such terms are necessary, definitions are provided in the text or in the glossary.

Remember, this book is designed to educate you, not to frighten you. Having IBD can be difficult, but you can learn to live with it — and to fight back. This book will help you do that.

1

The Normal GI System and IBD

Learning about a medical subject is much like learning about anything else. You have to start with the basics and build on that. To learn about a diseased bowel, you first have to learn about the healthy bowel.

The Normal Gastrointestinal System

The bowel is part of the gastrointestinal system, commonly referred to as the gastrointestinal tract, or GI tract for short. The GI tract begins at the mouth and ends with the anal canal. Most of it lies in the abdominal cavity, which is lined with a thin, transparent tissue called the *peritoneum*. The chief function of the GI tract is to digest food — to break it down into usable materials, then absorb them and eliminate the waste products.

When you eat, food goes from your mouth down your *esophagus* (the swallowing tube) into your *stomach*. Your stomach grinds the food and dilutes it. The resulting semiliquid gradually empties into the *small bowel*, or small intestine, which is 10 to 20 feet (3 to 6 meters) long and lies coiled in the middle of your abdomen.

The small bowel (also known as the small intestine) is made up of three parts. The first is the *duodenum*, which is just a few inches (centimeters) long. The next part, about 5 to 10 feet (1.5 to 3 meters) long, is the *jejunum*. This is where most of the food that we eat is digested and absorbed. The last 5 to 10 feet (1.5 to 3 meters) of the small bowel is the *ileum*. The juices produced by all three parts of the small intestine, as well as juices from the liver, gallbladder and pancreas, digest food and convert it into usable elements. Most carbohydrates (e.g., breads, potatoes, pasta) and proteins (e.g., meat, eggs,

9

The Gastrointestinal Tract

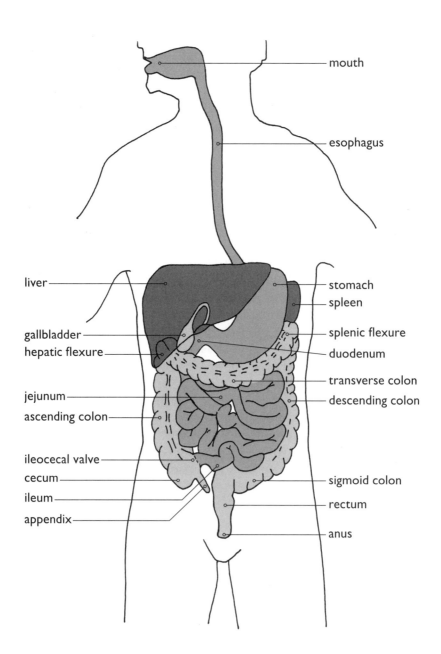

fish) are broken down and absorbed in the jejunum. Fats (e.g., butter, oil, margarine) are digested more slowly and require both the jejunum and ileum to be absorbed. Two things are absorbed mainly by the ileum: vitamin B12 and bile salts — an important point when people undergo surgery to remove this part of the small bowel.

The ileum runs into the *colon* low down on the right side of the abdomen. At the junction of the ileum and colon is a muscular thickening known as the *ileocecal valve*. It is not really a valve, but it opens and closes like a valve. This permits the small bowel to discharge its contents (mainly waste products) intermittently into the colon.

The colon, also known as the large bowel or large intestine, is much wider than the small intestine and is about 5 feet (1.5 meters) long. It too has different sections. The first is the *cecum*, which is a little cul-de-sac that lies below the junction of the ileum and the colon. The cecum probably does not have any specific function but, rather, is a remnant of evolution. The same may be true for the *appendix*, which projects from the cecum, although the appendix contains a lot of lymphoid tissue (part of the immune system) and this may be important.

Running upward from the cecum is the *ascending colon*. As you follow it, you will come to a sharp bend called the *hepatic flexure*. "Flexure" means bend; "hepatic" (from the Greek word for liver, *hepar*) indicates that the bend is at the liver. The segment of colon that runs from the hepatic flexure across the abdomen is called the *transverse colon*. The colon then turns sharply again at the *splenic flexure* (at the spleen).

The segment of colon that runs downward from the splenic flexure is called the *descending colon*. Following the descending colon is the *sigmoid colon*, named after the Greek letter *sigma* ("s") because the sigmoid curves frequently.

The *rectum* makes up the last section of the colon, although it is often treated as a separate entity. The *anal canal* is the outlet for the rectum. It is surrounded by the *anal sphincter*, a valve-like muscle that controls the passage of stool (waste matter) out of the rectum. The *anus* is the opening at the end of the canal.

These different sections of the colon do not have distinctive functions. However, the terms for the various sections of the colon allow more precise communication when describing a problem or a planned operation.

The colon has two main functions. One is to store waste material. The other is to absorb salt and water.

The terms "stool" and "feces" (pronounced fee-sees) refer to the material discharged from the rectum, whether it is solid or liquid. When the stool starts out near the cecum, it is brown water — it looks just like the water of a polluted river. When the stool comes out of the rectum, it is supposed to be a nice, neat package — not too hard, not too soft, not too big, not too small — about 1 foot (30 centimeters) long and sausage-shaped. As the brown fluid moves around the colon, the water is gradually absorbed by the lining of the colon so that the stool becomes more and more solid.

Many people think that most of a normal bowel movement is undigested food, but in fact, water makes up about 75 percent of a normal stool in the rectum. The GI tract is full of millions of different germs, mainly bacteria, mostly in the colon. They have a short life span and are constantly dying and being replaced by newly born bacteria; live and dead bacteria contribute about 8 percent to the bulk of the stool. Only about 4 percent comes from undigested food roughage (fiber). The lining of the whole GI tract replaces itself approximately every 72 hours, which means that a layer of dead tissue regularly "peels off"; this makes up about 3 percent of stool. The colon is always producing mucus, which is nature's lubricant, and this also ends up in the stool (1 percent). The remaining 9 percent is composed of a variety of substances.

When your rectum fills with stool, a message is sent to your brain telling it that the rectum needs to be emptied. If you sit on the toilet, the rectum will contract (squeeze), the anal sphincter will open, and the stool will be pushed out through the anal canal into the toilet. The normal process of digestion will have been completed.

Inflammatory Bowel Disease (IBD)

Inflammation — the word means "being set on fire" (from the Greek word for flame) — is a localized protective response that occurs when tissue is damaged or destroyed. Its purpose is to wall off, dilute or destroy an injurious agent. Acute inflammation is characterized by pain, heat, redness and swelling. Chronic inflammation is a less dramatic process. It may proceed without any of these features, yet it results in distortion — and sometimes destruction — of tissues, often leading to permanent scarring.

Inflammatory bowel disease is just that: disease in which the bowel becomes inflamed. By convention the term generally refers to only two diseases: ulcerative colitis and Crohn's disease. A few other diseases are sometimes included — microscopic colitis (including lymphocytic colitis and collagenous colitis), diverticulosis-associated colitis and Behçet's disease (more about those on pages 15–17).

One Disease, Two or More?

Some experts in the field have thought that ulcerative colitis and Crohn's disease are merely two forms of the same disease, perhaps because some people who initially have typical ulcerative colitis go on to develop features of Crohn's disease at a later date. It is extremely rare, though, for an expert to diagnose Crohn's colitis and then later change the diagnosis to ulcerative colitis. It is also extremely rare for both diseases to coexist in one person. Some experts think that the term "Crohn's disease" includes a group of diseases that are very similar but are distinguished by the fact that they respond to different kinds of medication. For example, some Crohn's patients respond best to antibiotics, whereas others respond best to steroids, and still others respond best to yet a different treatment.

When IBD is confined to the colon, doctors cannot always tell if the problem is ulcerative colitis or Crohn's colitis, and so tell such patients that they have "indeterminate colitis." This too has encouraged the perception of IBD as just one disease. In many cases, not being able to say which kind of colitis it is doesn't matter. Except when surgery is necessary, most treatments are the same for both ulcerative colitis and Crohn's disease.

Where Does Ulcerative Colitis Occur?

Ulcerative colitis occurs only in the colon. It always involves the rectum and, typically, it is continuous, that is, not confined to patches.

Some patients have inflammation just in the rectum (known as ulcerative proctitis). Others have it in the rectum and the sigmoid colon. Some have it in the rectum, the sigmoid colon, and the descending colon up to the splenic flexure. Others have it from the rectum around into the transverse colon. Some have it as far as the hepatic flexure. Yet others have it throughout the entire colon to the cecum.

Ulcerative colitis involves the rectum plus or minus the sigmoid in

Many Names: One Disease

It is common for different doctors to make up new names for specific diseases, especially those of unknown cause.

Other names for ulcerative colitis:
• idiopathic ulcerative colitis (idiopathic means "of unknown cause"),
• idiopathic proctocolitis,
• nonspecific ulcerative colitis.

Other names for Crohn's disease:
• ileitis, terminal ileitis ("terminal" refers to the terminus or end of the ileum — though most doctors avoid using the word "terminal" because people new to the disease may think the disease itself is terminal, that is, fatal);
• Crohn's disease of the colon/ileum/jejunum/duodenum/stomach/esophagus;
• Crohn's colitis, Crohn's ileitis, Crohn's jejunitis, Crohn's duodenitis, Crohn's gastritis, Crohn's esophagitis;
• regional enteritis, regional ileitis (old names, rarely used now);
• granulomatous ileitis/enteritis/colitis ("granulomatous" refers to a specific appearance under the microscope)—old names, rarely used now.

30 percent of cases, approximately the left half to two-thirds of the colon in 40 percent of cases, and the whole colon in 30 percent of cases.

Learning about medicine means accepting the fact that we can never say "never" and we can never say "always." Occasionally there are patients in whom ulcerative colitis is not continuous. What we see then is involvement of the rectum and some or all of the left side of the colon, plus a patch in the cecum, usually around the opening into the appendix. The patch near the appendix looks just like ulcerative colitis anywhere else. As you will see, patchy disease is typical of Crohn's disease; however, it is believed that those people with a patch of colitis around the appendix and typical ulcerative colitis elsewhere do in fact have ulcerative colitis.

In some patients with ulcerative colitis, the inner lining of the last few inches (centimeters) of the ileum becomes mildly inflamed. This inflammation is called backwash ileitis; it does not cause any symptoms or problems. We don't know why some patients get backwash ileitis and others don't.

Many people think that the word "colitis" is a short form for ulcerative colitis, but that's not the case. There are many kinds of colitis. If you have Crohn's disease in your colon, you have "Crohn's colitis."

Exactly What Is Inflamed in Ulcerative Colitis?
In ulcerative colitis, inflammation is usually confined to the inner lining of the colon, or mucosa. The surface of this inner lining becomes raw and bleeds easily, and looks a lot like scraped skin.

Where Does Crohn's Disease Occur?
Crohn's disease can occur anywhere from the mouth to the anus. Most commonly (45 percent) it occurs in the end of the ileum and the beginning of the colon (cecum plus or minus ascending colon). Second most commonly (35 percent) it occurs just in the end of the ileum. Third most commonly (20 percent) it occurs just in the colon. Here it may be patchy or continuous, and may or may not involve the rectum. In a few patients the jejunum, duodenum, stomach, esophagus or mouth is involved. For most patients with inflammation in these areas, the ileum or the colon, or both, are involved as well, but in a few people the disease is isolated in one or more of those locations. When Crohn's disease occurs in the mouth, it is almost always associated with Crohn's disease elsewhere in the GI tract.

Exactly What Is Inflamed in Crohn's Disease?
In Crohn's disease, the entire thickness of the bowel wall, from the inner lining (the mucosa) through the muscle layers to the outer lining (the serosa), is inflamed. In addition to swelling of the bowel wall, Crohn's disease causes swelling of the mesentery, a fan-shaped piece of tissue that supports and connects the small intestine to the back wall of the abdomen and contains the main intestinal blood vessels and lymph glands.

The "Other" IBDs
There are several conditions that are sometimes included under the label "inflammatory bowel disease": microscopic colitis, segmental colitis associated with diverticulosis and Behçet's disease.

MICROSCOPIC COLITIS

There are three forms of microscopic colitis, lymphocytic colitis, collagenous colitis, and mixed lymphocytic/collagenous colitis. These conditions are more common in women and more likely to occur in older age groups. People with microscopic colitis tend to have other autoimmune diseases.

Lymphocytic Colitis

In lymphocytic colitis, the colon appears perfectly normal at colonoscopy, but biopsies reveal an excess of white blood cells, especially those known as lymphocytes, indicating chronic inflammation. Stool tests for infection are negative, and routine blood tests and imaging of the GI tract are normal. People who have this form of colitis have chronic diarrhea, but they are not ill. Occasionally, this form of microscopic colitis is the forerunner of "real" IBD. Many people with this condition can be simply treated with antidiarrheal drugs such as loperamide (see Chapter 6). Some people will require more specific therapy with drugs used to treat ulcerative colitis. Surgery is not needed.

Collagenous Colitis

Collagenous colitis is another condition in which the colon appears perfectly normal at colonoscopy, and all routine tests are normal. However, unlike people with lymphocytic colitis, people with collagenous colitis can have all of the social inconveniences of "real" IBD — urgent, frequent, unpredictable bowel movements — but not the illness — things such as fever, loss of appetite and weight loss. Biopsies show a layer of collagen (which is like scar tissue) just below the inner lining of the colon. It is believed that this collagen layer acts as a mechanical barrier, preventing the absorption of water, which is one of the main functions of the colon. The result is watery diarrhea. (Most people who say they have watery diarrhea don't. A person who is used to having solid bowel movements will refer to any loose bowel movements as "watery." When I take a history from a person with diarrhea, I ask, "Is it pasty like toothpaste, mushy like porridge, or watery, as if you were passing urine from your rectum?" Truly watery *chronic* diarrhea is almost always due to a rare condition, such as collagenous colitis; there are many causes of acute, or short-term, watery diarrhea.)

Some people with collagenous colitis can be treated just with antidiarrheal drugs, such as loperamide (see Chapter 6). As with lymphocytic colitis, some people will need more specific therapy with the range of medications used to treat ulcerative colitis. *Unlike* lymphocytic colitis, many people with collagenous colitis will end up on steroids, and some will need surgery (an ileostomy, which is an opening of the ileum out to the skin, with or without colectomy —removal of the colon — or a pelvic pouch procedure) because of steroid dependency, or because medications don't work or stop working. If an ileostomy is created, the collagen layer disappears, but reappears if the ileostomy is closed. This is similar to what we see with Crohn's disease that is downstream of an ostomy (explained in more detail in Chapter 7).

SEGMENTAL COLITIS ASSOCIATED WITH DIVERTICULOSIS (SCAD)
With the widespread use of colonoscopy during the last 30 years, it has become clear that many people with diverticulosis involving the sigmoid colon have localized inflammation in the same area. This has many names in the literature, including "diverticulosis-associated colitis," but "SCAD" — segmental colitis associated with diverticulosis — is the most popular. This condition causes visible bleeding from the rectum more than it causes diarrhea. It is sometimes treated with 5-aminosalicylate (see Chapter 6), but it *can* get better on its own. The cause of this condition is unknown, and at times it may be difficult to distinguish it from Crohn's disease localized to the same area.

BEHÇET'S DISEASE
This condition is named after Hulusi Behçet, a Turkish dermatologist who first recognized the syndrome in a patient in 1924. However, like IBD, history tells us that this is a disease that had already been around for a long time. To be diagnosed with the condition, a person must have mouth ulcers (canker sores), of any shape size or number, at least three times in any 12-month period, along with two of these four hallmark symptoms:
• genital ulcers or swelling;
• one of various skin lesions;
• one of several kinds of eye inflammation;
• a pathergy reaction (a bump on the skin, at least 2 millimeters in diameter, 24 to 48 hours or more after needle prick).

However, people with this condition can also have a wide range of other signs and symptoms, many of which also occur in IBD. Some of these include joint pains or swelling, or both; stomach or bowel inflammation, or both; a tendency to form blood clots and a family history of the disease. The cause is unknown and the disease tends to wax and wane, just like IBD. The medications used to treat Behçet's disease are virtually identical to those used for IBD.

2

Who Gets IBD, and What Causes It?

Although there's still a lot that we don't know when it comes to who gets IBD and what causes it, researchers have collected many interesting statistics, which are helping us to put the puzzle together. In simple terms, here's what we do know: people are born with an inherited tendency to get IBD, then something in the environment — it might be a germ, or a food component or a chemical — comes along, and triggers or brings out the disease.

Who Gets IBD?

Inflammatory bowel disease can begin at any age. Most commonly it appears between the ages of 15 and 35, but it can appear for the first time at any age, from infancy to extreme old age. It occurs throughout the world, though it is much more prevalent in temperate climates than in tropical ones. It is found more often in developed areas such as North America, the United Kingdom, Scandinavia, and Western Europe than in developing countries. IBD has been very uncommon in Asia, even in the highly developed countries, but has become an increasing problem in Japan. Most studies report that IBD is more likely to occur in people of a higher socio-economic bracket. However, poorer people are less likely to seek treatment for their disease, so this may skew the studies. IBD may be a little more common in urban areas than in rural ones.

Is IBD More Common in Certain Population Groups?

IBD is more common in Jews than in non-Jews. But this applies only to Ashkenazi Jews, who are mostly from Eastern Europe — not to Sephardic Jews, who come from Spain and Portugal, or to Asiatic

Jews. IBD is much less common in blacks and Asians than in Caucasians. Asians are unlikely to have IBD if they live in the Far East, but develop it more frequently once they move to western countries. On the other hand, young Asians who are born in Britain are at a significantly higher risk of developing IBD than the indigenous European population.

Historically, IBD has been considered a "white" disease. However, it is clear that the reported rates for IBD in African-Americans have been steadily rising for several years. A multicenter U.S. study reported that African-American children and adolescents who are diagnosed with IBD are more likely to have Crohn's disease than ulcerative colitis, compared with non–African-Americans, and that the African-American children tend to present with their IBD at an older age, compared with their non–African-American counterparts. The reasons for these differences are not yet known.

In some parts of the world, males and females seem to get ulcerative colitis in equal numbers, but in most places, Crohn's disease is slightly more common in females than in males. One interesting study done several years ago suggested that left-handed people are twice as likely to get IBD (either form) as right-handers. A Danish study in 2003 confirmed earlier reports that Crohn's patients with pure colonic disease tend to be significantly older than patients with Crohn's in other areas of the intestine. Several groups have found that Crohn's patients of a young age at diagnosis tend to have more extensive disease, and more aggressive disease, with a significantly higher prevalence of upper gastrointestinal and ileal involvement than patients diagnosed later on in life.

What all this tells us is that the issue of who gets IBD, and why, is very complicated.

How Common Is IBD?

Many studies have been done to estimate the frequency of inflammatory bowel disease. Estimates of the number of cases in North America range from 10 per 100,000 to 1,000 per 100,000. Canadian researchers found that ulcerative colitis is present in an average of 194 of every 100,000 Canadians, with 11.8 new cases per 100,000 each year. Crohn's disease is even more common in Canada and is present in an average of 234 per 100,000 people, with 13.4 new cases per 100,000 each year. I use the term "average" because there are striking differences among the various regions of Canada. For example, in the province of British Columbia, on the west coast, the numbers are lowest, whereas in Alberta, which is the first province east of British Columbia, the numbers are among the highest in the country.

A U.S. study of nine million Americans, done by a group from several Boston hospitals and the Center for Inflammatory Bowel Disease in Boston, found that ulcerative colitis is present in an average of 238 per 100,000 people in the United States, while Crohn's disease is present in an average of 201 per 100,000 people. This group also reported on children under 20 years of age in whom they found ulcerative colitis in an average of 28 per 100,000 population, and Crohn's disease in an average of 43 per 100,000. As with the Canadian figures, I have used the word "average" because there are regional differences. For example, both forms of IBD were found to be less common in the southern United States, compared with the Northeast, Midwest and West.

Ulcerative colitis has been reported to be present in 58 to 157 per 100,000 population in northern Europe, while Crohn's disease prevalence ranges from 27 to 48 per 100,000 in northern Europe. Again, the range of figures reflects regional differences.

Is IBD on the Increase?
Several studies within the last couple of years have shown that new cases of IBD are on the rise in children, mainly in those up to 9 years old. In other age groups, the number of new cases of ulcerative colitis is stable, while Crohn's disease continues to increase. But, again, there are huge regional variations, which makes the accuracy of collecting this kind of information more difficult.

What Causes IBD?
We know a lot about IBD, but we don't yet know what causes it. Here are some of the factors that may play a role.

GENES AND IBD
There are many lines of evidence supporting the theory that IBD has a genetic component.

Families with IBD

It is important to realize that most IBD patients do not have any known relatives at all with IBD. But if a person has ulcerative colitis, there is a 6 to 10 percent chance of IBD in that person's siblings. If a person has Crohn's disease, there is about a 15 to 35 percent chance of IBD in that person's siblings. Within the extended family of someone with ulcerative colitis, there is a greater than expected chance of IBD, with ulcerative colitis being more likely than Crohn's disease. In the extended family of someone with Crohn's disease, there is again a greater than expected chance of IBD, with Crohn's disease being more likely than ulcerative colitis. The risk of the child of a person with IBD also developing the condition is thought to be about 5 percent. Remember that this means the child has about a 95 percent chance of *not* developing IBD. However, if both parents have IBD, the risk of IBD occurring in the children seems to be 35 to 50 percent.

Studies of identical twins have shown that if one twin develops Crohn's disease, the chance of the other twin developing it is 20 to 50 percent, usually within a few years. If one twin develops ulcerative colitis, however, the probability that the other twin will develop ulcerative colitis is much less, from zero to 7 percent. There are no reports of one identical twin having ulcerative colitis and the other having Crohn's disease. This tells us that these disorders have a similar but not identical genetic basis.

Specific Genes

Within the last few years, human gene research has provided us with some of the most exciting developments in medicine. In 2001, the first gene known to make people susceptible to Crohn's disease was discovered. Mutations (genetic changes) in this gene, known as NOD2 (also referred to CARD 15), located on chromosome 16, have been shown to predispose some people to Crohn's in the ileum, especially the form of the disease that causes a lot of scarring and narrowing. But not all patients with Crohn's disease have a mutation in NOD2. Such mutations have been found in one-quarter to one-third of Caucasian patients but are found much less often in Asians, Arabs and Africans with Crohn's. Moreover, a mutation in NOD2 does not necessarily mean that a person will develop Crohn's disease. NOD2 has been not been found to contribute to the development of ulcerative colitis.

Other genetic identifiers that have been discovered and confirmed by independent researchers include the IBD5 locus on chromosome 5q31, the IBD3 locus on chromosome 6p, the TNFSF15 gene (may only be significant in Japanese people), the IL23R gene and the AT-G16L1 gene. All of these are associated primarily with Crohn's disease. In comparison, little has been accomplished so far in the study of ulcerative colitis, although a Dutch research group has recently identified 10q26 as a locus for susceptibility to this condition. So, although gene studies have not yet determined the genes responsible for the *development* of IBD, discoveries to this point have revealed several genes that make people *susceptible* to IBD. Most of these genes have something to do with the ways our immune system responds to bacteria. When it comes to IBD genetic research, the terms to watch for are "GWAS" (genome-wide association studies) and "SNPs" (single nucleotide polymorphisms).

Blood Tests for IBD
There are numerous diseases in which the diagnosis is either confirmed or supported by one or more blood tests that are either specific or strongly suggestive. These tests are often referred to as markers. An antibody known as perinuclear anti-neutrophil cytoplasmic antibody (pANCA) is present in the blood of about 60 percent of people with ulcerative colitis and in a significant number of their relatives, even when those relatives do not have IBD. This antibody is found in the blood of 20 percent of people with Crohn's disease and a small proportion of their relatives and is not usually found at all in healthy families. Another antibody, anti-Saccharomyces cerevisiae antibody (ASCA), is present in the blood of about 60 percent of people with Crohn's disease and in the blood of some of their relatives, in 10 percent of people with ulcerative colitis, and in less than 5 percent of non-IBD patients.

Several other immune markers have been identified in the blood of some patients with IBD. Although the purpose of these antibodies remains unknown, identifying them in selected patients may be helpful when the diagnosis of IBD is difficult.

Intestinal Permeability
Another factor that may be inherited is increased permeability (leaki-ness) of the intestinal lining in people with Crohn's disease (see the section "Abnormal Immunity," below). Healthy people have an in-visible intestinal "barrier" that can prevent various substances from being absorbed. Canadian researchers have demonstrated that this barrier is "leaky" in people with Crohn's disease, so that substances that would not normally be absorbed may be able to enter the intes-tinal tissues and trigger inflammation. This "leakiness" is also found in some relatives of people with IBD.

Diseases Associated with IBD
Another line of evidence for the role of genetic factors is that certain other diseases occur more commonly in people with IBD. One of the best-known examples is the arthritic disease ankylosing spondylitis (discussed in Chapter 9). Canadian researchers have shown an asso-ciation between multiple sclerosis and Crohn's disease, and it is also known that people with Crohn's disease have a greater chance of hav-ing psoriasis.

The Future
Although we hear about new genetic discoveries in medicine every week, sorting out the genetics of IBD has proven to be a tough nut to crack. At present, genetic testing for susceptibility to IBD remains a re-search tool only, but it is expected that it will eventually become an im-portant part of clinical assessment of people with known or suspected IBD. Future research will also focus on the field of pharmacogenetics, which is the science of using genetic information to predict how well someone will respond to a particular drug or group of drugs.

While all this genetic information is important, we mustn't forget that it's widely accepted that there are environmental risk factors for IBD as well. "Environment" is being used in the broad sense here; the bacteria and other microbes in our intestines, plus any other chemi-cals or particles that we ingest, are part of that environment.

ABNORMAL IMMUNITY
Chapter 1 outlined the *digestive* functions of the GI tract. A second function, less well understood, is that of protecting the body against

potentially harmful infectious agents or chemical substances. The inner lining of the intestine (the mucosa) contains many types of immune cells that act as defenders to prevent infections. These immune cells release chemicals, called cytokines, which are responsible for coordinating the immune response to an infectious or chemical insult. Current research has demonstrated that an inappropriate or unbalanced release of these cytokines is involved in the abnormal immune response associated with inflammatory bowel disease.

As you've read above, our current understanding of why people develop IBD is that it is due to a combination of factors, including a hereditary tendency, exposure to one or more things in the environment and probably also other factors that we don't yet understand at all. Thus, it most likely takes the "perfect storm" combination of the right environmental trigger in a susceptible host to initiate the inappropriate release of inflammatory cytokines to produce what we recognize clinically as Crohn's disease and ulcerative colitis. The challenges now are to characterize the identity of these environmental triggers, as well as to understand the deregulation of the immune system in IBD.

Exciting recent research has implicated the bacteria that reside in the gut as one of the potential environmental triggers that may contribute to the development of IBD. Many researchers have looked at various possible roles for microbes in the development and perpetuation of IBD, and bacteria, especially our own, continue to be a hot topic in IBD research.

Billions of bacteria live in our gastrointestinal systems, mainly in the ileum and colon, where most IBD occurs. When we are born, we are "germ-free." As soon as we begin to take things into our mouths (and this starts in the birth canal), our intestines become home to many different bacteria and other microbes. Because we are not all exposed to the same environment, we do not all end up with the same microbial populations. Furthermore, it is likely that even people exposed to the *same* microbes will not all end up with the same populations, given inherited variations in immunity. We have come to understand that there are both "good" bacteria, which help us to maintain good health, and "bad" bacteria, associated with disease. It is widely believed that the more we learn about our internal "microbial community" (technically known as our microbiota), the better we will understand why things go wrong, and how.

The good bacteria are known as commensal organisms. In the past few years it has been discovered that the cells of the immune system, which include macrophages, B cells and T cells, exist in a fine balance with these good bacteria. Even though these commensal organisms closely resemble many infectious bacteria on a molecular level, our immune system has evolved so that it does not become activated by these good bacteria. Thus, it is said that our body is "tolerant" of these commensal intestinal inhabitants because the presence of these commensals in the gut does not result in inflammation. Although the precise molecular pathways that govern this tolerance are not fully understood, an emerging concept in IBD research is that failures in these mechanisms of immune tolerance to gut microflora contribute to the development of the disease. An example of this concept is what has been learned about the NOD2 gene.

Certain mutations in the NOD2 gene, as mentioned earlier, are associated with the development of Crohn's disease. NOD2 functions as a molecular sensor that detects the presence of bacteria. When NOD2 is working properly, it acts as a kind of immunological thermostat. NOD2 sets the immune system to a level of activity that prevents the commensal bacteria from crossing through the gut mucosa (inner lining) but also prevents the immune system from becoming fully activated and causing inflammation in response to the bacteria. It is believed that in some patients with Crohn's disease, NOD2 is unable to signal; in the absence of the "thermostat," this balance between the immune system and the commensal bacteria is lost. The bacteria are then able to cross through the gut mucosa and into the gut wall; this causes full activation of the immune system and the result is inflammation.

Since we know that less than half of the people with Crohn's disease have a mutation in NOD2, and since we know that a mutation in NOD2 does not mean that a person will definitely develop Crohn's, the NOD2 story reminds us how complicated a problem this is. This valuable discovery is instructive in showing us how disturbance of the commensal-host balance can result in disease, but it also demonstrates that much more research is required to discover other genes and factors involved in regulating this delicate equilibrium.

(Warning: this paragraph is for "budding immunologists" only!) In addition to having an abnormal balance between the immune system and the bacteria of the gut, patients with IBD have also been found

to have differences in the way their immune systems respond to particular stimuli. As we learned above, immune cells release chemicals, called cytokines, that are responsible for coordinating the immune response to various insults. The behavior of certain very important immune cells, named CD4+ T cells, has been shown to be altered in patients with IBD. Before becoming activated, CD4+ T cells are said to be "naive." Upon activation, these cells select one of many different "genetic programs" that will determine which cytokines these cells produce. Th1, Th2 and Th17 are just some of these genetic programs. All of the factors that influence the choice of program are not fully understood, but it is believed that the CD4+ T cell receives "instructions" from its environment as well as from other cells of the immune system to guide it down one particular genetic pathway. With a normal immune response, there is a well-controlled balance between all of these different genetic programs. In IBD, it has been found that this balance is lost and one or two of the genetic programs are favored. In Crohn's disease, it has been found that Th1 and Th17 cells predominate; in ulcerative colitis, there appears to be an excess of Th2 and Th17 cells. This loss of balance means that too much of certain cytokines, such as TNF-α, is produced; this overproduction fuels the intestinal inflammation. Many of the newer treatments for IBD attempt to rebalance cytokine production. Some of the biological drugs used to treat IBD (see Chapter 6), such as infliximab, adalimumab, certolizumab and golimumab block the TNF-α, which is produced by the Th1 T cells. Although this treatment is often beneficial, suppressing any part of the immune system can have undesirable side effects, as is discussed in Chapter 6. Furthermore, even though we know these targeted agents attempt to rebalance the immune response, we still have a very poor understanding as to why patients with IBD have an unbalanced immune response in the first place.

Clearly, an important theme in our current understanding of IBD is balance. A healthy gut is a finely tuned machine in which many balances are actively maintained. If one or more of these are disturbed, be it in the gut-commensal interactions or within the immune system itself, they contribute to initiating the inflammation that results in IBD. Understanding what tips the balance in the first place is the vital unknown. Below I describe two hypotheses that attempt to explain how the rapid advances in modern medicine of the last hundred years may have played a role in changing the balance in the gut environment.

The Hygiene Hypothesis

In the past 10 years, some researchers have come up with a new idea to try to explain why IBD is on the rise, especially in children. This idea is known as the hygiene hypothesis. The background for this concept is that our environment has become too "clean" (thanks to the development of better hygiene and the frequent use of antibiotics), and that this has resulted in a relative lack of early childhood exposure to various germs, such as bacteria and parasites. This is thought to increase susceptibility to certain diseases by affecting immune system

---

What About Stress?

The issue of stress and the gut is an important one. Many people in the general population (i.e., people who do not have IBD) have gastrointestinal problems when they are under stress, and this has led to an assumption that stress has a role to play in IBD as well. The condition known as irritable bowel syndrome (IBS) is a disorder in which people tend to have abdominal pain and irregular bowel movements without any intestinal inflammation. Many people with IBS have a considerable increase in their symptoms when they are mentally stressed. Everyone is familiar with the term "tension headaches," and people are not embarrassed to talk about them. But you don't hear a lot of people talking about their "tension vomiting" or "tension diarrhea" or "tension bellyaches," even though these are every bit as common. As with tension headaches, tension gut symptoms can occur in any pattern, from occasionally to daily.

Doctors used to think that IBD was caused by stress. There is no evidence for this, and it is no longer believed to be the case. Controversy still exists, however, about the possible role of stress as a precipitating factor in flare-ups in a person with preexisting IBD. Even if stress is a factor, it generally cannot be avoided, and the thought that a particular stress may cause a flare-up of the disease is in itself stressful. People with IBD can also have IBS, and no doubt the occurrence of both conditions in the same person helps to perpetuate the idea that stress causes IBD. The experienced doctor and the experienced IBD patient know that IBD can begin when things are going well or when they are going badly. Saying that IBD is a psychological illness suggests that, because of the kind of person you are, you are in some way responsible for the disease. This is likely to make you feel guilty, which can make you feel even worse. Remember, it's not your fault.

development. If you think this seems contradictory, you are correct. A simple way of stating this hypothesis is: If you are exposed to fewer infections, your immune system may not work properly, and you may get more infections or other illnesses that rely on a well-functioning, balanced immune response system. This leads us to the next idea.

The Old-Friends Hypothesis

A refinement of the hygiene hypothesis that overcomes its apparent contradiction is the old-friends hypothesis. This hypothesis modifies the hygiene hypothesis by proposing that T regulator cells (cells that regulate some of the activities of the immune system) can become fully effective only if they are stimulated by exposure to microbes that have a low tendency to make us sick, and which have coexisted universally with human beings throughout our evolutionary history. It's almost as if our immune system has to be trained to recognize friends and enemies. These concepts have been given more credibility by studies demonstrating the impact of infectious organisms, and helminths (parasitic worms) in particular, upon genes responsible for production of various cytokines. Dr. Joel Weinstock, an American researcher, has been a pioneer in so-called worm therapy. He has shown that some people with IBD improve substantially when they are "fed" certain worms that then temporarily live in the patient's intestine. But, like all other treatments affecting the immune system, this therapy has risks. Furthermore, this treatment is still experimental, and more research is needed.

IBD and Infections

Even though we believe that IBD can be triggered by a variety of infections, there is no convincing evidence that IBD is caused by one or more infections. But infectious colitis (which is caused by bacteria, viruses or parasites) and ulcerative colitis are similar, and Crohn's disease is strikingly similar to intestinal tuberculosis (which is caused by a bacterium).

Johne's disease is a Crohn's-like disease that occurs in a large variety of animals, but especially ruminants (such as cows and deer). The cause is a bacterium belonging to the tuberculosis family, known as Mycobacterium avium, subspecies paratuberculosis (Mycobacterium paratuberculosis, or just MAP for short). Some researchers have been strongly promoting the idea that Crohn's disease is caused by this bacterium.

They believe that milk and beef are the vehicles carrying the infection into the intestine. Despite their enthusiasm, most other experts in the field remain unconvinced, as this idea has been examined repeatedly over the last 30 years, with mostly negative results. Notwithstanding the inability to clearly link MAP with Crohn's disease, several centers for IBD have reported on treatment of Crohn's disease with a cocktail of drugs commonly used to treat tuberculosis. Unfortunately, results have been contradictory and confusing.

A more recent idea is that exposure to MAP early in life may predispose some people to Crohn's, although this idea is somewhat contradictory to the hygiene hypothesis, described on page 28.

Smoking and Crohn's Disease

Numerous studies conducted since 1987 have demonstrated that cigarette smoking is a risk factor for Crohn's disease, and female smokers are at a greater disadvantage than male smokers. Smoking also increases the likelihood that Crohn's disease will recur after surgery; giving up smoking soon after surgery makes a recurrence less likely. As well, smoking has been shown to greatly reduce the effectiveness of the drug infliximab (see Chapter 6). How smoking exerts these effects is unknown. However, the evidence is compelling enough that if you have Crohn's disease and you smoke, you should give it up. Paradoxically, nicotine seems to *protect* some people against ulcerative colitis.

As for second-hand smoke, the effects are similar. Passive smoking increases the risk of Crohn's disease in children but reduces the risk of developing ulcerative colitis.

Oral Contraceptives and IBD

Research on IBD among oral-contraceptive users is inconclusive. While the risk of developing IBD, especially Crohn's, seems to be increased, stopping the pill often makes no difference. Many gastroenterologists (physicians who specialize in treating diseases of the GI tract) consider it worthwhile for women with poorly controlled IBD to stop the pill temporarily to see what happens. If this is not possible, switching to a lower-estrogen pill is an alternative. Because the oral contraceptive remains one of the most effective forms of birth control, women should carefully consider the potential benefits and risks of stopping the pill or avoiding it altogether.

Other Lines of IBD Research

The more people there are trying to solve a problem, the more potential solutions will be offered. In the case of IBD, a broad range of concepts is being considered beyond that discussed above:

- A large body of experimental and clinical evidence suggests that a class of chemicals known as reactive oxygen metabolites may play an important role in the development of IBD. Some of these chemicals are classified as oxidants; others are referred to as free radicals. Some of the drug therapies used in IBD, such as 5-ASA (see Chapter 6), have potent antioxidant activity. However, much more work needs to be done to determine whether these chemicals have any importance in IBD.

- Nitric oxide is a short-lived molecule produced by the enzyme known as the nitric oxide synthase, in a reaction that converts arginine, an amino acid (amino acids are the building blocks of proteins) and oxygen into citrulline (another amino acid) and nitric oxide. Nitric oxide is involved in many disease processes. Despite an initial burst of enthusiasm, little hard evidence has been produced so far for any major role in IBD.

- It appears that having your appendix removed protects against ulcerative colitis. However, some researchers have suggested that this is true only if the appendix is removed before age 21. Conversely, appendectomy seems to increase the chance of developing Crohn's disease.

- From time to time, researchers have tried to link dietary factors to the development of IBD. Milk, cornflakes, a high intake of refined sugar, baker's yeast, and various other dietary constituents have been put forward as risk factors. To date, these hypotheses either have been disproved or have not been conclusively proved. Recently milk has reentered the picture, but as a vehicle for a tuberculosis-like bacterium (see IBD and Infections on page 29). It has been suggested that the significant components of food may be not the nutrients themselves but a variety of inert, inorganic, nonnutrient particles found routinely in our food. These include natural contaminants (soil and dust), food additives and anticaking agents. One idea is that these components may combine with bacterial particles, pass through a defective gut barrier and provoke inflammation.

So Where Does This Leave Us?

Our current understanding of the development of IBD is as follows. First, you must have a genetically susceptible subject. This person must then come in contact with an agent or substance that, through some defect in the normal intestinal defense system, is able to penetrate the intestinal wall. This sets up an inflammatory response. A defect (an imbalance) in regulating the inflammatory response must also exist so that, once the immune system is activated, a complex process is started that the body is unable to stop.

We still have no answer to the question of what causes IBD, but researchers in many countries worldwide are working hard to solve the mystery of these diseases. There is every reason to be optimistic and to believe that the causes of ulcerative colitis and Crohn's disease will eventually be found.

3

Symptoms and Signs

Symptoms are things that you can feel and describe to your doctor. Pain, poor appetite, nausea and diarrhea are common symptoms of IBD. Signs are things that you or your doctor can observe. Being pale, having a rash or passing blood into the toilet are all common signs of IBD. At times symptoms and signs are difficult to separate. If you have an itchy rash, the itch is a symptom and the rash is a sign. A diagnosis is easier to make with both symptoms and signs. This is why your doctor will frequently ask you many questions about a complaint. You can take a picture of a rash with your cell phone (but please don't take a picture of your toilet!), and e-mail it or show it to your doctor. The more information you give, the more accurate the diagnosis will be and the better the treatment.

Ulcerative Colitis
Symptoms of Ulcerative Colitis
The most typical characteristic of ulcerative colitis is bloody diarrhea: bloody diarrhea makes us think of ulcerative colitis, and ulcerative colitis makes us think of bloody diarrhea. There are always exceptions of course. Some people with this condition have bleeding without diarrhea, and some even have bleeding with constipation (particularly people with ulcerative proctitis). Mostly, though, it's bloody diarrhea.

Next to that, the most typical symptom of ulcerative colitis is the false urge: you get a feeling that you are going to have a bowel movement, but when you get to the toilet nothing or almost nothing comes out. Sometimes there's some gas, or some "wet" gas, or a little blood or even a bit of stool, but there is no reasonable amount of stool. The total number of trips to the toilet, for actual bowel movements *and* false urges combined, is one of the indicators of how severe an attack of colitis is. As a *rough* guide, 2 to 5 trips to the toilet in 24 hours indicate a mild attack of colitis, 5 to 10 trips indicate a moderate attack and 10 to 20 or 30 trips indicate a severe attack.

Closely related to the false urge is a symptom called tenesmus. You experience it as persistent pressure in the region of the anus; it feels like a constant false urge. It is usually not relieved completely (sometimes not at all) by passing gas or fluid or even solid feces.

Tenesmus is typically due to inflammation and spasm of the rectum. When a normal rectum is filled with stool, it sends a message to the brain that says, "Go to the bathroom and have a bowel movement." A healthy person responds by going to the bathroom but can also have the brain say to the rectum, "Not now — I'm busy." The rectum will relax and the urge to go the bathroom will disappear. When the rectum is inflamed, however, it is in spasm all the time. A rectum in spasm sends the same message to the brain as a full rectum. You may constantly feel you need to go to the bathroom even when there is nothing in the rectum, or just gas. The rectum does not accept the message "Not now — I'm busy." Even when you sit on the toilet, even if you have a bowel movement, this urge to pass stool is not completely relieved. The reason, of course, is that the rectum is still inflamed and therefore still in spasm, so the message from the rectum to the brain doesn't change very much.

Aside from bloody stools and frequent trips to the toilet, many people with ulcerative colitis experience crampy pain in the abdomen, low down on the left side, across the lower abdomen or across the upper and lower abdomen. Such pain, often described as squeezing, is usually followed by a trip to the toilet. Typically, the pain is relieved by passing stool or gas, or both.

Other symptoms that may be experienced by people with ulcerative colitis are reduced appetite, weight loss, lack of energy, fever, chills and sweats. These symptoms are either absent or mild in someone with a mild attack of colitis but can be dramatic in a severe attack.

Signs of Ulcerative Colitis

For most people with ulcerative colitis there are few signs of the disease other than blood in the stool. In some patients, the doctor can feel a fullness in the right lower quadrant of the abdomen. This is

IBD Look-alikes

Many medical conditions are characterized by diarrhea and crampy pain. Diagnosing inflammatory bowel disease means ruling these others out:

• Infections can mimic IBD: food poisoning or traveler's diarrhea (common causes are campylobacter, salmonella, E. coli, shigella), antibiotic-associated colitis (due to Clostridium difficile), yersiniosis, giardiasis, intestinal tuberculosis.

• Irritable bowel syndrome (IBS) can resemble Crohn's disease.

• Foods can cause chronic diarrhea: lactose, if you are lactose intolerant; caffeine; fructose; nonabsorbable sugars, such as sorbitol, mannitol, xylitol, maltitol and erythritol; a high-fiber diet.

• Drugs can cause chronic diarrhea: antibiotics, nonsteroidal anti-inflammatory drugs (NSAIDs), chemotherapeutic drugs and many others.

• Other IBD look-alikes include radiation enteritis after radiation treatment for certain cancers; ischemic (lack of blood flow) disease of the intestine; lymphocytic or collagenous colitis, or both; Behçet's disease; segmental colitis associated with diverticulosis (SCAD; see Chapter 1) and diversion colitis (see Chapter 7).

"They Thought I Had Appendicitis"

Some patients with undiagnosed small bowel Crohn's become ill suddenly and go to the hospital with severe abdominal pain. The attack is similar to acute appendicitis, and surgery may be necessary to make the correct diagnosis. The appendix is usually removed, whether it is normal or not. This is a good idea for the most part, as any future attacks will not be blamed on appendicitis.

because stool piles up in the ascending colon during an attack. The colon is extremely inefficient at emptying itself when it is inflamed. Even though you may go to the bathroom many times, you will usually pass only small amounts of stool, or even nothing.

Are People with Ulcerative Colitis Sick All the Time?

It is important to recognize that most people with ulcerative colitis are perfectly well between attacks. In any given person, attacks, or flare-ups, may occur frequently (every few weeks) or rarely (every few years). A person may have multiple flare-ups one year and then none for several years, or the attacks may follow any other irregular pattern that you can imagine. The average risk of a flare-up is about 10 percent per year. A small number of people with ulcerative colitis (about 5 percent) have what is known as chronic continuous colitis.

Crohn's Disease

Crohn's disease is somewhat more complicated than ulcerative colitis because it can affect different parts of the GI tract. The general symptoms are crampy abdominal pain, diarrhea and weight loss. Pain is most often felt around the navel or lower right part of the abdomen, or both. It is often associated with eating, and can begin during a meal, soon after or within an hour or so. A steady, dull ache in the lower right abdomen may also be felt. It is usually somewhat worse with activity, especially anything that jiggles the abdomen, such as jogging. Crohn's patients also suffer from a lack of energy.

Symptoms of Crohn's Disease of the Small Bowel

Some 70 to 80 percent of patients with small bowel Crohn's disease complain of crampy abdominal pain, diarrhea and weight loss. Many people quickly learn that they can avoid pain by avoiding food, and this is the main reason people lose weight. Occasionally, someone with small bowel Crohn's is troubled by constipation rather than diarrhea.

Symptoms of Crohn's Disease of the Colon (Crohn's Colitis)

The symptoms of Crohn's colitis are variable, depending on whether the disease occurs in the right side of the colon, the left side of the colon or the whole colon, and whether the rectum is involved. If the disease is primarily on the right side, you will have mainly cramps and diarrhea. If the disease is primarily on the left side or involves most of the colon, you will likely have cramps, diarrhea and some blood in the stool. If the rectum is involved, you will have symptoms similar to ulcerative colitis, with false urges (see the discussion on symptoms of ulcerative colitis on page 33).

Symptoms of Crohn's Disease of the Ileum and Colon

If you have both small bowel and large bowel disease, you may experience symptoms of the disease from either location, or from both. Crohn's of the ileum can flare up when the colonic disease is quiet, and vice versa.

Symptoms of Crohn's Disease of the Stomach or Duodenum

Many people with Crohn's disease in this part of the GI system have no symptoms, and the inflammation is discovered by chance. Of those who do have symptoms, over 90 percent have pain or discomfort in the upper abdomen (right side, middle or left side) that comes on during and soon after meals. Nausea or vomiting, or both, occur in about 30 percent of patients. Weight loss occurs in over 50 percent of people with symptoms as a result of the tendency to eat less in order to avoid the symptoms. Occasionally, Crohn's disease of the duodenum will mimic ordinary duodenal ulcer disease. In this situation, pain is more likely to occur when you have not eaten for a few hours, and the pain will be relieved by food.

In some people, Crohn's disease of the stomach or duodenum, or both, produces enough scarring that the outlet of the stomach into the duodenum, or the duodenum itself, becomes progressively narrower. You will be unable to eat a normal-sized meal, and you will have nausea, a prolonged full or bloated feeling in the upper abdomen after meals and, often, a decrease in appetite.

Symptoms of Crohn's Disease of the Esophagus

This is so rare a form of Crohn's disease that it is not possible to say what the typical symptoms are. Most people are likely to experience chest pain behind the breastbone, usually when they swallow. The esophagus may become narrow; some solid foods may get stuck on the way down; if you are having this problem, tell your doctor.

Symptoms of Crohn's Disease of the Mouth

Just like esophageal Crohn's, this condition is rare, making it difficult to say what is typical. However, if you have Crohn's disease and you get large, painful sores in your mouth, this is more likely to be Crohn's disease than the much more common canker sores that occur in both the general population and people with IBD. If you are having this problem, tell your doctor.

Symptoms of Crohn's Disease of the Appendix

Appendicitis due to Crohn's disease may precede symptoms of Crohn's disease elsewhere in the gastrointestinal tract. However, Crohn's disease of the appendix can be present without symptoms in someone who has symptoms of Crohn's disease elsewhere.

As with garden-variety appendicitis, the usual symptom is a sudden onset of pain low down on the right side of the abdomen. Slow healing or development of a fistula (an abnormal connection between two organs, or between a hollow organ and the skin surface) after an appendectomy is a clue.

Signs of Crohn's Disease

Unlike those with ulcerative colitis, many people with Crohn's have specific signs that, together with the symptoms, point quite strongly to the disease. About 25 percent have an easily felt area of swelling, most commonly in the lower right part of the abdomen. This is much more distinct than the vague fullness that can be felt in some people with ulcerative colitis. The swelling is often the size of a small grapefruit, and often as firm. The area is usually tender, and the tenderness can be anything from mild to extreme. If it is mild, the swelling is usually the result of inflamed intestine and surrounding tissues and enlarged lymph glands. If there is a marked tenderness, the swelling is usually due to an abscess (boil). In this case the overlying skin may be red, and it may look stretched. In some people, generally those with moderate tenderness, the swelling is due to a combination of swollen tissues and an abscess. In someone thin, the swelling in the abdomen may be visible.

Another common sign of Crohn's disease is perianal disease (disease around the anus). This occurs in about 25 percent of cases and usually takes the form of a fistula, with or without one or more abscesses. Some people have very swollen tags of skin around the anus. This finding is quite characteristic of Crohn's disease. Many people who develop hemorrhoids but don't have IBD get skin tags, but swelling of these tags is minimal.

Is It Crohn's or IBS?

The main alternative diagnosis to Crohn's disease is irritable bowel syndrome (IBS). However, people with IBS rarely lose weight. Early in the onset of symptoms of Crohn's disease there may not be weight loss, and this may delay the correct diagnosis. Here's a case in point.

A 21-year-old woman developed crampy pain around her navel and mild diarrhea with three to four mushy bowel movements a day. The crampy pain and diarrhea came mainly after meals. She was otherwise well and had never been sick before. When the symptoms persisted for two weeks and became slightly worse, she went to see her family doctor. He examined her abdomen, said it was normal, and told her she probably had IBS. No X-rays or blood tests were performed. The woman was reassured.

Four weeks later the symptoms were still present and somewhat worse. The woman was now having four to six bowel movements a day, and occasionally got up at night to have them. She had lost 10 pounds (almost 5 kilograms). She decided to go see her mother's family doctor. The physical examination, blood tests and an X-ray of the abdomen were normal. Again she was told that she probably had IBS. When asked if she was nervous, she said that she was. (Anyone having cramps in the abdomen and unpredictable diarrhea for 6 weeks is bound to be a little nervous!) She was offered a tranquilizer. She tried it, but it just made her feel dopey and did not change her symptoms.

Four more weeks passed. By this time she had lost 20 pounds (almost 10 kilograms). She went back to her own doctor. He arranged for a CT scan of the abdomen, which revealed Crohn's disease in the ileum. The woman was promptly referred to a gastroenterologist and treatment was started, with good results.

In the past, this was a very common sequence of events. Statistics in the 1970s indicated that the average time it took for a diagnosis of Crohn's disease to be made once a patient began complaining of symptoms was 3 years. Since some people were diagnosed quickly, this means that in other people the delay was much longer. Over the past 40 years, much more attention has been given in medical schools to IBD. As a result, doctors now think of it sooner, make the diagnosis more quickly and start treatment faster. In many cases, this prevents the patient from losing a lot of weight and becoming seriously ill.

Are People with Crohn's Disease Sick All the Time?

People with Crohn's disease are more likely than those with ulcerative colitis to experience persistent symptoms between flare-ups. But many people are ill only intermittently. As with ulcerative colitis, attacks may occur every few weeks, months or years. A person may have multiple flare-ups in one year and then none for several years, or in any other irregular pattern that you can imagine. The average risk of a flare-up is about 30 percent per year.

4

How Is IBD Diagnosed?

Physicians have a growing arsenal of tools to aid them in diagnosing inflammatory bowel disease. However, before we get to those diagnostic aids, remember that the first steps in assessing patients are the history and the physical exam. In many cases of IBD, the doctor can make the diagnosis with that information alone, and the tests described below simply confirm the diagnosis and clarify the extent of the problem.

Ulcerative Colitis and Crohn's Colitis

Ulcerative colitis is initially suspected from symptoms — frequent, urgent trips to the bathroom and bloody diarrhea — and the typically raw or scraped appearance of the rectum when the doctor examines it with an endoscope. During the endoscopy, the doctor will usually take a biopsy (tissue sample) to confirm the diagnosis, and may also arrange to have stools sent to a lab to check for infections that mimic ulcerative colitis.

Crohn's colitis may produce exactly the same symptoms as ulcerative colitis, although visible bleeding is less common, and is often diagnosed in the same way.

SIGMOIDOSCOPY

A patient suspected of having ulcerative colitis or Crohn's colitis will undergo either a sigmoidoscopy or a colonoscopy. These days, most patients will have a flexible sigmoidoscopy ("-oscopy" means to look into; to look into the sigmoid colon is sigmoidoscopy). This involves passing an instrument through the anus into the rectum, and then into the sigmoid colon. The instrument may be a colonoscope, a flexible sigmoidoscope (which is really just a shortened colonoscope) or a rigid scope (used much less now than in the past, but still used by some physicians, mainly in the office, to get a quick diagnosis). The procedure allows the physician to view the mucosa of the bowel.

COLONOSCOPY
In a colonoscopy (looking into the colon), the doctor examines most or all of the colon. Colonoscopy can be used to diagnose IBD and to determine how much of the colon is inflamed. During the procedure, the end of the ileum can also be examined in most people; this is useful, since the end of the ileum, plus or minus the right side of the colon, is the most common location of Crohn's disease. Colonoscopy can be used as well to check for precancerous conditions or cancer itself (see Chapter 10). The procedure is usually done on an outpatient basis. Even if you have diarrhea, the colon often needs to be cleaned out for colonoscopy. Sedation is often given to relax you and minimize discomfort. In some people it is not possible, for technical reasons, to pass the colonoscope all the way around the colon. In others, strictures (areas of narrowing) may prevent passage of the instrument. In such cases, other options include a CT scan with a small amount of dye inserted into the rectum, or a virtual colonoscopy (this is usually a CT colonography, but can also be an MR colongraphy).

Preparation for Colonoscopy
Cleansing the colon for colonoscopy requires that the colon is flushed out with a large volume of fluid. This can be achieved in one of two ways: a large-volume prep or a concentrated prep.

For many people, the safest and most effective way is to drink a colonic lavage solution — commonly known as a large-volume prep — a solution containing electrolytes and polyethylene glycol (PEG for short). But for many, this type of preparation has a bad reputation. There are two main reasons for this. The first is that the manufacturers

---

The technologies used to obtain pictures of the various parts of the body are collectively known as medical imaging. Techniques include ultrasound, Doppler ultrasound, CT (or CAT) scans, MR (or MRI) scans and PET scans. Ultrasound and MR scans have the advantage of not using radiation.

of these products instruct the patient to drink 250 milliliters every 10 minutes. If you do this, you are going to drink 4 liters in less than 3 hours. This is difficult to do. You will feel very bloated and full, until you start to have bowel movements. Many people also become very nauseated, and some will vomit. The fact is that it is not necessary to drink the fluid so quickly. I tell my patients to drink the 4 liters over 4 to 8 hours, or even longer, if they wish. This makes a *big* difference. The second reason why many people don't like this prep is because they don't like the taste of the product. Ask your doctor what the various products taste like, and choose the one that appeals to you the most. It's not going to taste *good* but hopefully you'll be able to put up with it.

However, some people can't or won't drink a large-volume prep. The main alternative is to drink a concentrated product — usually supplied as two packets of powder, to be dissolved — which literally sucks the needed water out of your body and into your bowel. Some people find this easier, but it is vital to understand that you must drink a lot of clear fluids (apple juice, ginger ale, consommé, tea) to replace what has been sucked into the intestine. You should aim to drink at least 2 liters of clear fluids. If you don't do this, you may become dehydrated, which can have serious consequences. This method of cleaning out your bowel sounds a lot easier, and more pleasant, than drinking a large-volume product, but many people become quite nauseated soon after drinking the second packet and then don't drink enough and become dehydrated.

The most commonly used preparations are electrolyte solutions (large volume), sodium picosulfate (small volume), magnesium citrate (small volume), or a combination of these. All can cause nausea, vomiting, abdominal fullness and crampy abdominal pain. Sometimes, these side effects are so severe that the person is unable to continue taking the preparation. Through trial and error, most people find at least one preparation that they can tolerate. Additional information on two of these agents can be found in Chapter 6.

Risks of Colonoscopy
Although colonoscopy is a very useful procedure, and while it is fairly safe, there are some risks. All of these risks are uncommon; I have not

included actual percentages because different doctors quote different numbers, often based on their own experience, in combination with the figures in the literature. Here are the ones I outline for my patients:

- Drug reaction: any of the various preps can cause an allergic reaction. The most likely is an itchy rash. The nausea and vomiting that may occur with the preps are common side effects and are not allergic. The medications used to sedate you for the procedure can also cause an allergic reaction.
- Bruise of the colon wall: you will have pain for a few days following colonoscopy, but tests will likely be normal. No specific treatment is needed, and, like all bruises, this gets better by itself.
- Tear of the colon wall: this usually results from excessive stretching of a portion of the colon, sometimes in an area of adhesions (see Chapter 7). Tears usually require surgical repair.
- Cautery perforation (burning a hole in the colon wall): this can occur during the destruction or removal of polyps. Some small polyps can be removed without cautery, removing this risk. Most cautery perforations can be managed without surgery. You will be given antibiotics, and you will not be allowed to eat or drink for a few days.
- Bleeding: whenever a polyp is removed, bleeding may occur. If it's a problem at the time of removal, the bleeding can be stopped with an injection into the area, or with cautery introduced or with tiny clips. Bleeding can occur up to 2 weeks after removal of a polyp, when the scab falls off. If you start bleeding, the best thing to do is to go to the closest ER. The bleeding can stop on its own, but a colonoscopy may have to be done to stop the bleeding. Some people bleed enough that a blood transfusion is necessary. Surgery is very rarely needed.
- The risk of missing something; this is a different kind of risk than all the others in this list. Colonoscopy is a very effective procedure, but it is not perfect. No matter how clean your colon is, and no matter how carefully your doctor looks, there is always a risk that something will be missed, occasionally something very important, such as an early cancer. The main reason for this is that "driving" through the colon is not like driving on a straight road, where you can constantly see both sides of the road. The colon is more like a winding country road, with blind curves and dips.

AIR-CONTRAST BARIUM ENEMA

Most people with ulcerative colitis or Crohn's colitis have the extent of their disease determined by colonoscopy, but it can be estimated with an air-contrast barium enema, which is an X-ray of the colon. After the bowel has been appropriately cleansed, a small, short tube is inserted into the rectum, and air and a suspension of barium sulfate (an inert substance easily visible on X-rays) are blown into the colon and multiple pictures are taken. The technique shows details of the inner lining of the colon, which is irregular instead of smooth in people with colitis. The usage of barium enemas has decreased steadily in recent years, mainly replaced by colonoscopy, with CT scans as back-up, and, just recently, by MR exams. But family doctors who suspect either ulcerative colitis or Crohn's colitis may still send you for one. If you are allergic to CT contrast (the intravenous dye used with many, but not all, CT scans), a gastroenterologist or surgeon may also want you to undergo a barium enema. In some people it is not possible, for technical reasons, to pass a colonoscope all the way around the colon. In other people, strictures may prevent passage of the instrument. Although many such cases are evaluated with a CT scan or an MR study, a barium enema may also be used in those situations.

CT (OR CAT) COLONOGRAPHY

This is a specialized form of CT scan. This technique is used primarily to look for polyps in people who are unwilling or unable to have colonoscopy, or who have had an incomplete colonoscopy. At the time of writing, a prep (similar to that for colonoscopy) is still necessary, but it is expected that this will change in the future. Air is blown into the colon to inflate it (this can be painful), then a very rapid CT scan is performed. So far, this technique is not very good for polyps less than about one-third of an inch (1 centimeter) in diameter but is better than colonoscopy for finding polyps above that size. If polyps are found, a colonoscopy is usually the next step.

So far, CT colonography has played only a minor role in IBD. While it can be useful, most, if not all, of the information obtained can be seen with ordinary CT scanning. The latest innovation in imaging is the combination of CT and PET scanning.

PET/CT COLONOGRAPHY

This combined technique has recently been reported to provide a non-invasive way of assessing IBD during a disease flare when, in some patients, colonoscopy is more risky. This sounds promising, but further study is needed.

Crohn's Disease of the Small Bowel

Small bowel Crohn's disease is suspected when a person suffers abdominal cramps and diarrhea, with weight loss, for more than 2 weeks. A mass of swollen tissue that can be felt in the abdomen strongly increases the doctor's suspicion. Abscesses or fistulas around the anus are even stronger indicators.

The way that Crohn's disease is diagnosed often depends on who first investigates the diagnosis. If it's your family doctor, it is likely that you will have an imaging study of some kind — for example, an ultrasound, CT scan or MR. If you are referred to a gastroenterologist or a surgeon for diagnosis, it is more likely that you will have a colonoscopy, probably followed by a CT scan. Advantages of colonoscopy for diagnosis of Crohn's disease are that (1) disease may be found in people whose X-rays might be normal; and (2) abnormal areas can be biopsied to confirm the diagnosis, or to discover that another disease, and not Crohn's, is present. Disadvantages of colonoscopy are that (1) many people with Crohn's have it just in the ileum, and because the disease frequently causes narrowing of the intestine, it may not be possible to pass the scope from the colon into the ileum — this may suggest the presence of Crohn's, but is not good enough to confirm the diagnosis; and (2) it is sometimes very difficult to take the colonoscopy preparation if a person is unwell and having abdominal pain and frequent bowel movements. Even if colonoscopy is completely successful, imaging of some kind is important, to allow your doctor to determine if there's any obvious Crohn's disease in the small bowel, beyond the reach of routine endoscopy.

There are several ways to use X-rays to diagnose Crohn's disease in the ileum. For all of these tests, the only preparation is to have nothing to eat or drink after midnight the night before the test. If the test is in the morning, try not to eat any solid food for at least 2 hours before bedtime.

CT SCAN OF THE ABDOMEN AND PELVIS, CT ENTEROGRAPHY
AND CT ENTEROCLYSIS

In a CT scan (also known as a CAT scan), a computerized X-ray machine very rapidly takes hundreds of pictures of "slices" of your body, in different planes. The computer then recreates the desired images of your intestine, which can be viewed on an ordinary monitor. For most of these studies, the patient is given a drink of a dye that helps outline the inner lining of the intestine and, also, an intravenous dye, which highlights details in the wall of the intestine and in the surrounding tissues, such as the mesentery, which supports and connects the small intestine to the back wall of the abdomen.

The CT enterography is a CT scan dedicated to examination of the small intestine. It can "kill two birds with one stone" because it still provides information about all the other structures in the abdomen, just like a regular CT scan. But even a plain CT scan can demonstrate many of the features of Crohn's disease, including the presence and location of the abscesses and fistulas that occur as a complication of Crohn's disease (see Chapter 9).

In some cases, the doctor or the radiologist may wish to perform a special type of CT enterography, in which a little plastic tube is inserted through the nose, down the esophagus, into the stomach, and then into the duodenum. The contrast material is injected into your intestine through the tube, instead of you drinking it. This is called CT enteroclysis. This method may show more detail than a tubeless study. But a lot of people don't like the tube; you can ask to have some local anesthetic sprayed into your nose first to reduce the discomfort.

MR ENTEROGRAPHY

Over the course of their disease, Crohn's patients often require repeated imaging of the abdomen. Because multiple CT scans involve significant amounts of radiation, there is starting to be a shift to using MR, which is safe for most people.

BARIUM SMALL BOWEL SERIES AND BARIUM SMALL BOWEL ENEMA

A barium small bowel series (also known as a small bowel follow-through) was the standard small bowel exam before CT scanning was available; it is still done, but much less often. You are given two or three large glasses of barium sulfate suspension to drink. X-rays are taken at set intervals until the barium reaches the colon. At that time, the radiologist usually takes pictures of the end of the ileum. In most people with Crohn's of the ileum, the disease is obvious.

With the barium small bowel enema (also known as small bowel enteroclysis) method, a tube is inserted into your small bowel, as described on page 46. Barium is injected through the tube and monitored as it progresses through the small bowel. The main advantage of this technique is that it is sometimes more accurate than a small bowel series. As with the small bowel series, it is still done, but much less often.

CAPSULE ENDOSCOPY (THE PILLCAM®)

This method for examining the small intestine has generated much excitement. You swallow a capsule about the size of a large vitamin pill. The capsule, which is eventually expelled, contains a battery, a light, a video chip and a transmitter. Images of the inner surface (mucosa) of the small intestine are transmitted to a recorder on your belt. The main application of this test is to look for obscure causes of gastrointestinal bleeding. It can also be used to find Crohn's disease that is not demonstrable by other methods. Risks are few, but the capsule can get stuck at a stricture, causing obstruction, which can lead to emergency surgery. This risk is greatly reduced by using a pretest dummy capsule, which gradually dissolves if it gets stuck. Your doctor will know if it gets stuck because you will develop symptoms of obstruction. The capsule is expensive, and it's unnecessary for most people with Crohn's. So far, it has not been very useful for examining the colon, but this is changing.

ENTEROSCOPY

This is an endoscopic procedure used to examine the small intestine. There are currently three techniques: push enteroscopy, single-balloon and double-balloon enteroscopies.

Crohn's disease of the jejunum or the ileum, or of both, is generally diagnosed using one of the medical imaging techniques described on page 49 (except for the very end of the ileum, which is often accessible with the colonoscope). Occasionally, enteroscopy is used to examine the jejunum and, sometimes, the ileum, directly. Your throat is frozen with a spray, intravenous sedation is given, and a scope is passed through your mouth, down the esophagus, through the stomach, and into the small bowel to make — or possibly exclude — a diagnosis of Crohn's disease. Although enteroscopy is useful, the simplest form, push enteroscopy, enables doctors to visualize only the first 3 to 4 feet (about 1 meter) of the jejunum, and most small bowel Crohn's is in the ileum, well beyond the reach of the usual enteroscopic exam. The single-balloon technique allows doctors to get farther down, but usually still not to the ileum, where most Crohn's is found. The double-balloon technique allows examination of the whole small intestine in some people, but it takes many hours and requires heavy sedation. Some people even have to be admitted to the hospital for this procedure.

Crohn's Disease of the Esophagus, Stomach and Duodenum

ESOPHAGOGASTRODUODENOSCOPY

Crohn's disease of the esophagus, stomach or duodenum is generally diagnosed by an esophagogastroduodenoscopy. This procedure involves passing a scope through the nose, or into the mouth and down the throat, after appropriate freezing or sedation, or both. Often referred to as EGD or OGD, the procedure is generally painless, or nearly so. Biopsies, which you don't feel, may be taken. Sedation is given to relax you if you are anxious about the procedure, and you may fall asleep, but it is not a general anesthetic.

UPPER GI SERIES

Occasionally, Crohn's disease of the esophagus, stomach or duodenum will be diagnosed with a barium X-ray known as an upper GI series. You drink a barium sulfate suspension (generally flavored, which helps a little), and a radiologist takes pictures.

Ultrasound

Although using sound waves (ultrasound) to examine the bowel does not allow a specific diagnosis to be made, it can sometimes show thickened bowel when someone is too ill to undergo routine diagnostic testing. Thickened bowel has several causes, but one of the more common ones is Crohn's disease. Ultrasound can also be used to diagnose certain complications of IBD, especially abscesses and fistulas within the abdomen or pelvis. In women, trans-vaginal ultrasound may also be used to diagnose complications of Crohn's. As well, ultrasound can be used to evaluate the response of Crohn's disease to drug therapy.

Which Is Better: Ultrasound or CT Scan?

Ultrasound is believed to be perfectly safe. A CT scan involves radiation. Gas in the bowel can greatly interfere with the transmission of sound waves, so if a patient has a bowel obstruction or some other reason for having a lot of gas in the bowel, a CT scan will be better than ultrasound.

Magnetic Resonance Imaging (MR, MRI)

This technology has proven useful in assessing some people with Crohn's disease, especially those with abscesses or fistulas, or both, particularly in the perianal area. This can be very helpful in surgical planning in some people. MR enteroclysis, a method of examining the small intestine, is still in development, and its place in the evaluation of Crohn's is not fully established. At the time of writing, MR colonography has a limited role in assessing the disease. If this imaging is being done, you will need to take a prep similar to that for colonoscopy. At the time of the study, your colon is filled with water via a tube inserted into your rectum; the images are then obtained.

One of the attractions of MR is its safety for most people. But there are serious risks in certain people; you should be asked to complete a questionnaire before the test is booked, to determine whether you are at any risk.

Leukocyte (White Blood Cell) Scan

This test shows areas of intestinal inflammation by identifying concentrations of white blood cells. It doesn't hurt, and there are no risks. The test is popular in some IBD centers, particularly for children. However, it is not specific for Crohn's disease and has no advantages over other methods of diagnosis in the vast majority of cases.

5

Diet and Nutrition

Once the diagnosis of inflammatory bowel disease has been confirmed through tests, and other diseases have been ruled out, the question becomes how to treat it. One of the areas of greatest interest to many people with IBD is diet. They often experiment with changes in diet, sometimes even before they have received medical advice. People with Crohn's disease often discover that they feel better if they don't eat any solid food. Unfortunately, this worsens the weight loss many experience. Some mistakenly believe that greasy or spicy food should be avoided, but then their diet becomes boring. This can lead to eating even less food and losing more weight.

When someone is ill and needs drugs or surgery, or both, sometimes maintaining adequate nutrition becomes an afterthought. But good nutrition is always desirable for those with IBD, as it is for everyone. Knowing what good nutrition means is important. If your doctor can't answer all your food-related questions, you can get advice from a dietitian. Be aware that in some countries the term "nutritionist" can be used by anyone; ask your doctor to refer you to someone who is properly trained.

Most people with IBD can eat a perfectly normal or near-normal diet most of the time. But when you are ill, sometimes avoiding certain foods is recommended, or a liquid diet is prescribed. If you know you are eating poorly, you should take a one-a-day multivitamin and

There is a widespread public belief, popularized by some books and the Internet, that there are specific diets for Crohn's disease and ulcerative colitis. This is not true.

mineral preparation (tablet or liquid). Don't use products that contain amounts above the recommended daily allowance or other substances. I advise my patients to buy a standard house-brand product at a large chain pharmacy and take one dose a day.

Common Dietary Restrictions in IBD

Lactose

Lactose, commonly known as "milk sugar," is a sugar found in dairy products. Some people with IBD experience less pain, diarrhea and gas if they restrict lactose in their diet.

In the inner lining of the small intestine, we all have a variety of enzymes (proteins that digest — break down — other chemicals). One of these enzymes is lactase, and its function is to digest lactose. When lactose is acted on by lactase, it is broken down into two simpler sugars: glucose and galactose; both are rapidly and easily absorbed through the small intestine into the bloodstream.

As long as you have enough lactase enzyme for the lactose you take in, there is no problem. All the lactose will be digested, and the resulting glucose and galactose will be absorbed. But if you don't produce enough lactase, only some of the lactose will be digested. As the undigested lactose travels down the small intestine, it causes water to be drawn into the intestine by osmosis. This water is held in the intestine and may produce cramps. The extra fluid in the intestine may also cause loose bowel movements (diarrhea).

When this undigested lactose reaches the colon, it *is* digested, not by us, but by the bacteria we all have there. The process is known as fermentation. When lactose is fermented by bacteria, it is broken down into an acid and lots of gas. The gas can cause a bloated feeling, pain in the abdomen and an excess passage of gas from the rectum. The acid can cause anal burning.

WHAT IS LACTOSE INTOLERANCE?

The symptoms — bloating, pain, diarrhea, gas — that result from a failure to digest lactose are referred to collectively as "lactose intolerance." Some people use the term "lactase deficiency." It really doesn't matter which term you use. The fact is that if you ingest more lactose than your small intestine can handle, you will have some or all of these symptoms. Despite popular belief, this is not an allergy. Most people with lactose intolerance can handle a certain amount of lactose; the amount is different in different people.

WHO BECOMES LACTOSE INTOLERANT?

As we get older we gradually lose some of our lactase enzyme and thus are less able to process lactose-containing food. This doesn't happen to everyone, but it happens to many people. It is not serious; it is a nuisance. Of course, it's unpleasant to have abdominal pain, diarrhea or a lot of gas, but it's important to remember that, in this case, it's not dangerous.

Lactose intolerance is more common in those of African and Asian descent than in Caucasians. As mentioned in Chapter 2, IBD is more common in Jews than in non-Jews. As it happens, lactose intolerance is also more common in Jews than in certain other ethnic groups. Lactose intolerance can occur in conjunction with IBD, but it is not the cause of IBD. It is also not an allergy. There is some evidence that

Lactose Intolerance

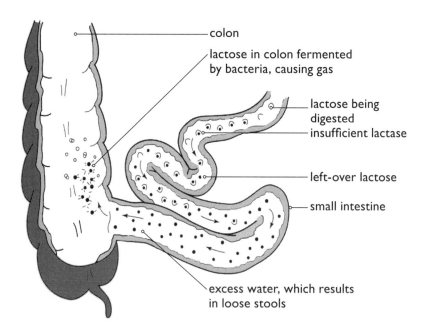

- colon
- lactose in colon fermented by bacteria, causing gas
- lactose being digested
- insufficient lactase
- left-over lactose
- small intestine
- excess water, which results in loose stools

lactose intolerance may be a little more common in people with IBD than in other people, but this is not definite.

People who are not known to have lactose intolerance may experience it for the first time at the onset of their disease. It is worthwhile to avoid lactose to see if it makes a difference. If it does not, then there is no point in avoiding it, because dairy products are a good source of nutrients and energy, both of which are important when you are ill. If avoiding lactose *does* make a difference, remember that the problem may be temporary. It may last for just a few days, though it can last several months. Once your diarrhea is under control, it is worthwhile experimenting every so often to see whether you need to continue to avoid lactose. Even if you can't resume taking the amount of lactose that was in your diet before you developed IBD, you should try adding

---

Are You Lactose Intolerant?

Some doctors diagnose lactose intolerance by doing a lactose tolerance test. The most practical and direct way to determine lactose intolerance is to vary the amount of lactose in the diet.

Let's compare a couple of examples.

A young woman developed ulcerative colitis. She was treated with medication but was also told to avoid all milk and milk products. Her disease came under good control. She was advised to stay on the low-lactose diet indefinitely. She consulted another gastroenterologist because she was unhappy about having to avoid dairy products and was told she should gradually increase her intake of milk and milk products. She was able to resume her usual habit of a glass of milk a day and cheese three to four times a week. There was no evidence of lactose intolerance.

A middle-aged man was referred to a physician for a second opinion because he had persistent diarrhea with his Crohn's disease despite taking several medications. He said he had never tried any dietary restriction. He was in the habit of having cold cereal with milk every morning, cheese two or three times a week in a sandwich, yogurt occasionally, and ice cream frequently in the summer. He was advised to stop all milk, cheese, yogurt and ice cream for 1 week, then report back. Before restricting his intake of lactose, he was having 5 to 10 watery bowel movements a day with an excessive amount of gas. One week later he reported that he was having 3 to 5 bowel movements a day with much less gas. Because of this improvement, he was referred to a dietitian for advice on a strict lactose-free diet. Two weeks later, he was having 1 or 2 normal bowel movements a day. Clearly, he was made completely better by eliminating lactose from his diet.

back the things you miss the most to see whether you really need to avoid them.

Remember that you cannot harm yourself by eating lactose-containing foods when you are ill with IBD, even if you have lactose intolerance. You may go to the bathroom more, you may have more abdominal discomfort and you may have more gas, but this does not mean your disease has gotten worse. Obviously, it may be difficult to tell what is going on if this happens, however, and the simple solution is to remove lactose from your diet temporarily.

Lastly, the lactase enzyme is believed to be inducible in some people. What this means is that your body *may* increase its production of lactase if you regularly exceed the amount of lactose that you can tolerate.

TRYING A LOW-LACTOSE DIET OR LACTOSE-FREE DIET

If you want to avoid lactose to see if that reduces cramps and diarrhea, consider trying a low-lactose diet — no milk, no cheese, no yogurt, no ice cream, no *obvious* milk products (without reading the labels). If your diet contains few milk products to start with, or if avoidance of milk and milk products produces only a partial benefit, it may be worthwhile trying a lactose-*free* diet to see whether further benefit can be achieved (see Appendix 2).

Once you have established the degree of benefit you can achieve with a lactose-free diet, you can add back foods containing small amounts of lactose, such as margarine, breads, cereals, baked goods and processed meats. You can then move on to try foods that contain greater amounts of lactose, such as cottage cheese and other cheeses,

---

Hidden Lactose

Many foods contain lactose but are not so labeled. A typical example is processed meat. Lactose is a cheap filler and is used liberally in hot dogs, for instance, to make them larger. Whey may be listed as an ingredient — it contains lactose, which may not be listed. Commercial gravies usually contain lactose because it can increase the volume of the gravy considerably. Some breads are made with milk; one way to avoid them is to buy bread at a kosher Jewish bakery, where milk is not used in preparing bread. As well, many pills contain lactose. People with a marked lactose intolerance may experience symptoms if they take them.

sour cream and yogurt. If you still don't have any significant symptoms, try adding back even more foods. You may discover that your lactose intolerance was temporary and that restriction is no longer needed. Another possibility is that your lactose intolerance is mild, in which case you will experience excess lower bowel gas, but little or no diarrhea.

There are several things to keep in mind when it comes to lactose:

- An average North American adult meal plan provides about 25 to 30 grams of lactose a day.
- The main sources of dietary lactose are milk and milk products; 8 ounces (250 milliliters) of milk contain 12 to 13 grams of lactose.
- Fermenting (aging) cheese converts most of the lactose to lactic acid, which is not a problem for your body. However, other fermented dairy products, such as buttermilk or sour cream, contain significant amounts of lactose.
- Lactose is added in small amounts during processing of many food and drug products. Lactose is present if the label states the addition of milk, milk solids, cheese flavor, whey, curds and some margarines, unless specifically labeled as nondairy.
- Lactic acid, lactalbumin, lactate and casein (milk protein) do *not* contain lactose.

Having a Good Calcium Intake If You Are Lactose Intolerant

If you're on a low-lactose diet, you may not get enough calcium, vitamin D, protein and energy (caloric intake). There are ways to have dairy products while avoiding most or all lactose:

- Buy lactose-free milk and ice cream. Pure lactase enzyme, which predigests much of the lactose, is added at the dairy. Some people find that the milk and ice cream taste a little sweeter than usual.
- Take lactase tablets just before and while eating foods containing lactose. Lactase enzyme is commercially available in both liquid and tablet form. The tablets are especially handy when you are eating in a restaurant, as you may not know which foods contain dairy products or added lactose.
- Eat aged cheeses. Aging cheese reduces the amount of lactose in it because aging involves adding bacteria to cause fermentation. Old cheddar contains very little lactose and can be eaten comfortably

by most people with lactose intolerance. Those with mild lactose intolerance can generally eat cheeses that are less aged, such as medium cheddar.

- Eat yogurt made with live bacterial culture. All yogurts are made with bacteria, but labeling identifies those with live (active) bacteria. The bacteria used produce lactase enzyme and release it. Thus at least some of the lactose in the yogurt can be digested.

IS EXTRA CALCIUM NEEDED IF YOU ARE LACTOSE INTOLERANT?
If you're trying a low-lactose diet, there is no urgency about taking calcium pills. The body can easily do without the lost calcium for weeks, even a few months. The body controls the blood calcium level the way a thermostat controls the temperature in a house. If the blood calcium level is a little low, the body extracts calcium from the bones. Of course, this can make the bones soft and more prone to fracture. But other factors influence the strength of the bones, such as exercise, the amount of vitamin D in the diet and exposure to sunlight, which leads to the formation of vitamin D in the skin.

Many adults develop osteoporosis as they get older. The use of steroids such as prednisone to treat IBD increases the risk. It is well recognized that calcium can be added to the skeleton easily up to the age of 35. After that age it becomes more difficult. Providing enough calcium to prevent further deterioration seems to be effective, although medications may also be needed to treat osteoporosis, or to try to prevent it (see Chapter 6).

Once you have established what level of lactose you can tolerate, having a registered dietitian assess the amount of calcium in your diet is useful, or you can do it yourself. (See the calcium intake assessment in Appendix 3.) You then need to review your conclusions with your doctor, so that it can be determined whether you need a supplement, and how much. You may need a bone density test to determine whether you need to go on a specific medication to help strengthen your bones.

Even if you're not lactose intolerant, you may be wondering if you should take calcium supplements. This topic is discussed in more detail in Chapter 6.

Fiber or "Roughage"

Fruit, vegetables and grains are considered essential ingredients of a healthy, well-balanced diet. Some of these foods have a laxative effect, and this may be undesirable when you are in the midst of a flare-up of IBD. These foods can also result in excessive gas, which may be particularly bothersome during a flare-up.

Two chemicals in fruit are likely to act as laxatives: sorbitol and fructose. Sorbitol is present primarily in prunes, pears, cherries, and peaches. It is also used as a sweetener in many kinds of gum, in some mints and in some liquid medications. We are unable to digest sorbitol and have a limited ability to absorb fructose. We can handle some of either one without getting a laxative effect, but if an excess (which differs from person to person) of one or both is taken in, it acts just like lactose in a person with lactose intolerance. Like unabsorbed lactose, both cause water to be drawn into the intestine by osmosis, and this leads to loose stools. And just like unabsorbed lactose, both are broken down in the colon by bacteria, releasing excessive gas. In addition to sorbitol, many gums, candies and other processed foods contain one or more of the sugars mannitol, xylitol, maltol, maltitol and erythritol, which can have the same effects as sorbitol.

Many vegetables and grains are a natural source of gas. The gas is produced when bacteria digest complex-carbohydrate residue in the colon. An enzyme product called alpha-galactosidase can predigest the fiber in these foods before it reaches the colon. The breakdown products do not produce gas. Alpha-galactosidase may be effective in reducing gas from peas and beans, nuts and seeds, grains and cereals, and a variety of vegetables. (A detailed list is available from the manufacturer.) It is used by mixing a few drops in with those foods that may produce gas, or by taking tablets with your meals. It is available in most pharmacies. People who are allergic to penicillin may also be allergic to alpha-galactosidase, because it is taken from a mold, just like penicillin.

Someone having a flare-up of IBD may well be more comfortable avoiding fruits and vegetables. Many people with IBD can return to eating these foods between flare-ups. However, others always have a degree of diarrhea and recognize that they are better off without these foods, good as they may be.

It is perfectly all right to experiment with different fruits and vegetables to see if you tolerate some better than others. Some people know that they have to avoid foods that contain sorbitol but that they will have no difficulty with other fruit, for instance, some berries.

People who have small bowel Crohn's disease with a narrowing (stricture) in the small intestine may have particular difficulty with fibrous foods because the stricture is fixed in size and cannot get wider, no matter how hard the intestine tries to push fibrous foods through. These people may get crampy pain when they eat some fruits and vegetables. Cereal fiber, such as bran, may not cause a problem for small bowel Crohn's patients because bran can change shape and be squeezed through the narrowed areas. Bran may have to be avoided, though, because it is a potent laxative. It also produces troublesome gas in some people.

Restricting fruits and vegetables necessarily means a decreased intake of minerals (potassium and iron) and vitamins (A, C and folate. The solutions are to increase your intake of bananas, citrus juices, tomato juice, ketchup and brown sugar (for potassium and vitamin C); increase your intake of meat (for iron and folate); increase milk and milk products (lactose-free if you are lactose intolerant) and liver (for vitamin A); eat whole-grain cereals (for fiber) and avoid only coarse fibers (celery, apple skins) and large seeds. An alternative is to take a one-a-day multivitamin and mineral tablet. If that's your choice, I recommend you take a standard (nothing extra added) house-brand tablet from a large chain pharmacy.

MEAT

Some people with IBD think they feel better if they avoid meat. Certain bacteria in the colon act on meat residues and produce hydrogen sulfide gas. There is some evidence that this is bad for the health of the cells in the lining of the colon, and that this may be a factor in aggravating colitis. But this is controversial, and meat is a good source of protein and iron.

FAT

Some patients with small bowel Crohn's disease do have to reduce the amount of fat in their diet, if the last 3 feet (about 1 meter) or more of the ileum is severely diseased, or has been surgically removed or bypassed (see Chapter 7). Fat absorption is very likely to be decreased and diarrhea will result or, if already present, will likely be aggravated. This results in a loss of energy intake (and probably a loss of weight).

How Can a Patient on a Low-Fat Diet Compensate?
If you are on a low-fat diet, can maintain an acceptable weight and are not bothered by the fat restriction, there is nothing you need do. But if you need to gain weight or you would like to use fat for salad dressing or cooking, there is a manufactured food product you can use. It is known as MCT, which stands for medium-chain triglyceride. Many nutritional products contain MCTs, but there are only two products in which MCTs make up all or most of the fat.

The first is MCT oil. This is a pure liquid oil product derived from coconut oil. Many people take it as they would any liquid medication. It can also be mixed with fruit juices, used on salads and other vegetables, incorporated into sauces or used in other cooking and baking. One tablespoon (15 milliliters) provides 115 calories. The second product comes as a powder and must be mixed with water before use.

Foods or Food Components That Can Cause Diarrhea
Diarrhea may be caused or worsened by certain foods:
• Lactose (milk sugar): see Appendix 2.
• Fiber: vegetables, fruit, grains.
• Fructose (fruit sugar) (see Appendix 4): While fructose does not require any digestion, we have a limited ability to absorb it. If you take in more than your small intestine can handle at any particular time, the extra fructose will cause gas and diarrhea via the same mechanism as unabsorbed lactose.
• Nondigestible, nonabsorbable sugars (sorbitol, mannitol, xylitol, maltol, maltitol, erythritol). These are sugars that we cannot digest or absorb. They are present in most chewing gums (sugarless or not), many confections (such as candies) and some processed foods. You must read labels to detect these. Some of them, e.g., sorbitol, occur naturally in certain foods. They cause gas and diarrhea via the same mechanism as unabsorbed lactose.
• Caffeine: Caffeine is present in coffee, tea, cola, cocoa and chocolate. If you think this is a cause of diarrhea for you, decaffeinated products should be okay. If this is not a problem for you, there is no need, and no benefit to your IBD, in avoiding caffeine.

Many people with IBD wonder if they should take vitamin and mineral supplements on a regular, ongoing basis. For a detailed discussion of this topic, see Chapter 6.

Large amounts of these products can cause drowsiness or confusion in individuals with advanced cirrhosis of the liver, so caution should be exercised.

LIQUID DIETS

Clear Fluid Diet

Sometimes it is necessary to avoid all food except for clear fluids. In certain situations this can improve your symptoms dramatically — particularly if you have small bowel Crohn's disease and especially if the symptoms are due to a partial small bowel obstruction.

If you are in the hospital and have not been allowed to eat or drink anything, clear fluids are wonderful, even enjoyable for a day or two. After that, this diet gets pretty boring, not to mention that it is very poor nutritionally. It supplies only 400 to 600 calories per day, with about 135 grams of carbohydrate, 8 grams of protein and no fat. A person weighing 150 pounds (about 70 kilograms) needs at least 1,500 calories, 60 grams of protein and a small amount of fat each day. So it is important for both you and your doctor to remember that you should not be on clear fluids for more than a few days, unless there's no choice.

Full Fluid Diet

A patient doing well on a clear fluid diet may move to a full fluid diet. A typical full fluid diet provides 1,100 to 1,300 calories a day, and usually contains at least 165 grams of carbohydrate, 40 grams of protein and an equivalent amount of fat. If lactose intolerance is not a problem, this diet is certainly a great improvement over a clear fluid diet, though it does not include enough energy or protein for most people recovering from an illness or an operation. If you are lactose intolerant, a full fluid diet cannot be used, since many of the foods in it contain dairy products. In fact, if you subtract the dairy products from the full fluid diet, you are pretty well back to clear fluids. Furthermore, a lot of older people don't like sugar or milk products. This is important to remember, because older people are more vulnerable to various illnesses and complications, especially if they are malnourished.

Why Restrict All Solids?

The purpose of restricting solids is to eliminate most residue (indigestible matter) from the diet. This is important for people with small bowel Crohn's disease with partial obstruction or an acute flare-up, but also for some people with fistulas (due to Crohn's disease or as a complication of surgery) or people with short bowel syndrome (see TPN, on page 65). But as we've seen, restricting solids in the diet can result in an inadequate intake of energy and some nutrients.

Elemental Diets, Polymeric Diets and Modular Products
A wide range of specialized nutritional products is available to insure adequate nutrition for people who must stay on a fluid diet.

An elemental diet is one in which all nutrients are in their simplest forms. The carbohydrate is present as glucose; the protein is present as amino acids; any fat that is present (usually very little) is in the form of long- or medium-chain triglycerides. These components are mixed with all the necessary vitamins, minerals and trace elements. In concept, the elemental diet is predigested. In reality, however, the fat supplied requires some digestion. These products are generally available in a powdered form and must be dissolved in water and used within 48 hours. Truly elemental diets are rarely used these days. When they are used, it is via tube feeding, as very few people can tolerate the taste.

Polymeric diets contain complex chemical forms of the various nutrients. For example, carbohydrate may be present in the form of corn syrup; protein is often in the form of casein (milk protein, and nothing to do with lactose); fat may be in the form of corn oil. Other ingredients may be added to make these diets more palatable. Most of these products are marketed in liquid form in cans or boxes. A few of the polymeric diets are very low in fat. Some come in powdered form and must be mixed with water before use. The canned or boxed products generally have a shelf life of approximately 2 years. However, once a can or a box has been opened, it must be refrigerated, and it will stay good for only 48 hours. The majority of these products are lactose-free.

Modular products supply one particular nutrient. The medium-chain triglyceride (MCT) product to replace fat is an example of a modular product. Protein powder is another popular modular product.

High-Glutamine Products
Glutamine is a nonessential amino acid. "Nonessential" means that the body is able to produce it, in comparison with "essential" amino

acids, which must be taken in because the body is unable to manufacture them. During physical stresses such as surgery or severe illness, the body may need more glutamine than it can produce.

Research has shown that glutamine is an important nutrient for the jejunum. This has led some manufacturers of nutritional support products to promote high-glutamine products. But there is little evidence that glutamine is beneficial to the ileum, where the majority of small bowel Crohn's disease occurs, and there is no conclusive evidence that high-glutamine products offer any special benefit to people with Crohn's disease generally.

When Are Liquid Diets Used in IBD?
ULCERATIVE COLITIS
There are times when someone with ulcerative colitis does not feel like eating much, but is willing to drink. Since most ordinary fluids are filling without supplying a lot of energy, liquid diet products can prove very useful. It is also possible to have high-energy, nutritious liquids that are not manufactured. The two best examples are milkshakes and eggnog; they are high in both energy and protein. However, because they also contain a lot of lactose, some people with lactose intolerance cannot use them. If someone with ulcerative colitis *can* eat a reasonably normal diet, there is no advantage to using specialized products. Nutritional therapy alone is not a treatment for ulcerative colitis.

CROHN'S DISEASE
Unlike for ulcerative colitis, nutritional therapy alone is an effective treatment for Crohn's disease, especially when the disease is active in the small bowel. In adults, these diets are most often used by patients who want to avoid using steroids to treat the problem, by doctors who want their patients to avoid steroids or by people who want to stop using steroids but have been unable to do so. Most people who go on a liquid diet will be able to reduce steroids without having a flare-up. A substantial number will be able either to stay off steroids or to use a reduced dose when the liquid-diet course is finished and a regular diet has been resumed. Although it was initially thought that the diet had to be elemental, it has been conclusively shown that polymeric diets are just as good. There is still some controversy about whether all polymeric diets are equally effective. Liquid-diet therapy

can be as effective as prednisone, the steroid most commonly used for Crohn's disease, though it doesn't work as often as prednisone does. (See Chapter 6 for more information on steroids.)

How Do Liquid-Diet Products Work?

So far, we don't know *exactly* why liquid-diet therapy works. However, since these products are sterilized and most regular food is not, it is very likely that certain bacteria, or components of bacteria, aggravate the inflammation of Crohn's disease (see Chapter 2). There is also some evidence that simply making sure you are properly nourished can be beneficial for Crohn's disease.

Does Liquid-Diet Therapy Work for Everyone?

No treatment for Crohn's disease works for everyone, and this is no exception. This type of therapy works particularly well in people with small bowel Crohn's disease. It works much less often in patients with Crohn's disease of the colon.

Tube Feeding

There are three situations in which liquid diets are taken by tube:
- when a patient cannot drink enough to achieve an energy goal because they cannot find a product that is palatable;
- to reduce or prevent side effects such as nausea or diarrhea; and
- to administer a product that is meant to be given by tube, usually because it is simply undrinkable because of its taste or some other feature.

The tube is inserted into the stomach through the nose. This sounds unpleasant, but the tubes are small and soft, and generally they are well tolerated. Although the liquid diet can be dripped in through the tube using gravity alone, it is often administered using a pump. For some people, controlling the rate of delivery with the pump is important; for others it is not. Battery-operated pumps allow people to move around both in and out of hospital during the process.

When following a liquid diet, it's important that you know how to calculate your nutritional needs. You'll find details on this on page 199, How to Use an Enteral Diet.

Some adults will do almost anything to avoid being tube fed. Children, on the other hand, adapt well to this form of treatment (see Chapter 8).

Advantages of Liquid-Diet Therapy

If nutritional therapy is to be used, one of the greatest advantages of a liquid diet is that the majority of people can stay out of hospital while using it. It is also a safe means of treatment, provided the doctor or dietitian instructing you is familiar with it. You do not have to stay home. You can go to work, school or anywhere else. As long as you are able to consume the desired amount of energy per day (see Chapter 12), you really have no restrictions whatsoever on your activities.

Disadvantages of Liquid-Diet Therapy

Liquid-diet therapy does, however, have several disadvantages. One is cost. Of course, when you are not eating a regular diet, that cost saving must be taken into account. But generally it does not cancel out the cost of the specialized diet. Unfortunately, insurance companies rarely pay for these products, claiming they are food and not treatment. Some government health plans do pay, but for specific groups only.

A second disadvantage is taste fatigue. Many people find they can take these products for a few days but get bored with the taste after that. Even when people can handle these products for longer, most prefer one flavor. This again leads to taste fatigue. Using a variety of clear fluids, flavorings or recipes helps. Water-based products, for example, can be made into a slush or even frozen.

Ultimately, you will have to stop the liquid-diet therapy. Even if you feel perfectly well on a liquid diet, only after you stop the diet will you and your doctor know if anything has really been accomplished. As soon as you go back to regular food, your previous symptoms of Crohn's disease *may* immediately reappear.

Additional problems for some people on liquid diets include nausea, a perpetual feeling of unpleasant fullness, abdominal cramps and frequent or loose stools. Obviously, some of these side effects can easily be confused with the Crohn's disease that is being treated. You can reduce these side effects by sipping the product slowly; take 30 to 60 minutes for one can or box, especially during the first few days. Although some people have one small bowel movement every few days, one to three loose movements a day should not be considered a problem.

Can You Have Regular Food While on a Liquid Diet?

Liquid-diet products do not provide enough water, so you must take a certain amount of clear fluids every day. I tell my patients to take the liquid diet when hungry and clear fluids when thirsty. You can also have clear fluids to combat taste fatigue, provided that you still achieve your daily energy goal.

How Long Should You Stay on a Liquid Diet?

There are no hard-and-fast rules about how long to stay on a liquid diet. I tell my patients that they must fulfill two conditions before they can go back to regular food. First, they have to take the liquid diet for a minimum of 2 weeks. Second, they must feel perfectly well for a minimum of 1 week. If a patient feels much better but not perfectly well and has not improved further for a week, then I compromise and accept partial improvement. Generally, the maximum period I prescribe a liquid diet for is 8 weeks, but it can be taken indefinitely.

Total Parenteral Nutrition (TPN)

In the term *total parenteral nutrition* or TPN, "total" refers to providing a nutritionally complete diet; "parenteral" means that the diet is given by a route other than the GI tract. In the late 1960s it became possible to feed people high-energy diets intravenously. This meant that people with Crohn's disease could avoid food, improve and still receive adequate nutrition.

In the 1970s this was a popular treatment for the disease. However, in the late 1970s and through the early 1980s it became increasingly obvious that most such people could be equally well treated with oral liquid diets. As awareness of the risks and expense of TPN has grown, more and more patients are treated with liquid diets. For some, nutritional therapy is a combination of a liquid diet and parenteral nutrition (known as PPN or partial PN). Although most people receive TPN in hospital, some receive it at home (known as HPN — home parenteral nutrition).

Today, TPN and PPN are reserved mainly for patients who are acutely ill, such as those with severe colitis or toxic megacolon (see Chapter 9); for patients who have chronic bowel obstruction and are awaiting surgery; and for people with short bowel syndrome, especially those who simply don't have enough remaining small intestine for maintenance of adequate nutrition. Many of these people can't or won't eat enough to maintain adequate nutrition.

Occasionally, people with Crohn's disease need prolonged temporary or even permanent PN to maintain adequate nutrition or adequate body water balance, or both. Others require a long period of nutritional buildup prior to surgery and can't or aren't allowed to eat enough to achieve this. Still others — fortunately, not very many — have had most of their small bowel removed surgically and don't have enough intestine left to absorb all nutrients (short bowel syndrome). Such patients receive HPN, or home parenteral nutrition. This may be TPN or PPN, depending on the amount of intestine left. Just as with home tube feeding, those on HPN become quite knowledgeable and self-reliant

---

The Gottschall Diet (the Specific Carbohydrate Diet)

The Specific Carbohydrate Diet was designed in the 1920s by an American, Dr. Sidney Haas, and then popularized by biochemist and cell biologist Elaine Gottschall. The cornerstones of the diet are to reduce intake of complex carbohydrates and completely remove refined sugar, gluten (a protein in barley, rye and wheat) and starch from the diet. It has been claimed to benefit people with a variety of unrelated conditions, including irritable bowel syndrome, Crohn's disease, ulcerative colitis and autism. One of the claims made by proponents of this diet is that the lining of the gastro-intestinal system in people with these diseases overproduces mucus, resulting in an injury, which in turn causes reduced nutrient absorption. Not only is there no evidence for this idea of mucus overproduction, but also mucus is a naturally occurring substance, produced by the healthy intestine, and acting as nature's lubricant. There is no reason to think that mucus is harmful; in fact, we know that the mucus layer has protective qualities. Lastly, there is no reason to believe that mucus, even if overproduced, would cause any problems with digestion or absorption of foodstuffs.

The idea of the diet is to keep the good bacteria well balanced and to starve out the bad. The diet forbids certain foods, suggesting various substitutes. This diet is not part of mainstream therapy for IBD. Nevertheless, many patients, especially those who aren't doing well and are frustrated, try it. If you read the claims of benefit with this diet, remember that, in most studies in IBD, 30 percent of patients have a measurable positive response to placebo (something that contains no medicine but may provide a positive effect because the patient *believes* that they are receiving a treatment). *It is important to be aware that most people lose a lot of weight on this diet. If you are planning to go on this diet, discuss it with your doctor first.*

about administering the IV diet and maintaining the IV site. Some hospitals have HPN programs to teach the technique.

The main advantages of TPN are that it can prevent or reduce nutritional deterioration in seriously ill patients, and it can be a virtual lifeline to people unable to get proper nutrition because of an inadequate amount of intestine.

The main disadvantages are that TPN is highly specialized and expensive. Furthermore, the need to have foreign material (the IV line) in the body constantly puts the person at risk of blood infections and blood clots — both potentially life-threatening complications. Another risk is the possible development of liver inflammation; this can lead to cirrhosis of the liver, which in turn may cause liver failure, and even a need for a liver transplantation.

Unnecessary Dietary Restrictions in IBD

Some people need to restrict their diet all the time, some need to do it some of the time and others can always eat a perfectly normal diet. Many people, however, restrict their diets unnecessarily. Sometimes the doctor has imposed these restrictions, but in other cases they are self-imposed.

Is It Necessary to Avoid Fried or Spicy Foods?

For the vast majority of people with IBD, there is absolutely no need to avoid fried or spicy foods. You may be underweight, particularly if you have been ill, and fat is an excellent source of energy. Fried foods not only taste good but will help you regain lost weight. Spices improve taste, which helps to increase food intake.

I am not suggesting you eat a high-fat diet all the time, since fat may increase the risk of heart disease and other diseases. But when you're trying to regain weight, it is generally harmless to eat an increased amount of fat. When I have a patient who is having trouble gaining weight after a flare-up of IBD, I often suggest high-fat, high-energy foods such as bacon and eggs, potato chips, various fried foods, cake and ice cream.

Adverse Effects of Unnecessary Restrictions

If you avoid two or three foods because you think they may increase your symptoms, it's generally not a problem. But if you have a long list of foods that you avoid, it's likely that your disease is active and needs specific therapy. Avoiding a large number of foods usually decreases your appetite because your diet becomes boring. Eating less, of course, reduces the amount of energy you take in, which leads to weight loss. Someone with active disease is likely already underweight, and losing more weight is undesirable.

Four Steps to Avoiding Self-imposed Dietary Restrictions

For many people with IBD, there is already enough adversity; give yourself a break, and don't make things worse than they are:

- Avoid restrictions based on hearsay. When I ask patients why they are avoiding certain foods, they sometimes tell me that they "heard somewhere" that such a food could cause symptoms. Friends and relatives are rarely a reliable source of medical or nutritional advice.

- If you think you've found a relationship between certain foods and certain symptoms, discuss your theory with your physician before permanently limiting yourself.

- If you're older, and especially if you live alone, put more effort into preparing meals. Otherwise your diet will be boring, you'll eat less and you'll lose weight. Older people, particularly when they are ill, need balanced meals.

- Many people avoid foods they can recognize in their bowel movements because of the mistaken belief that there is something wrong with their digestion. Humans cannot digest (break down) many of the components of dietary fiber. If you eat corn, you will see corn in your stool. The same is true for a large variety of skins, seeds and other fibrous foods. This is normal. Get your head out of the toilet!

Remember, dietary restrictions should be discussed with your doctor or a registered dietitian. You can experiment yourself but do not maintain any long-term restrictions without letting your doctor know.

6

Drugs, Probiotics and Other Treatments

Before getting into the details of drug therapy, I want to remind you of the old saying "A little learning is a dangerous thing." Knowledge is good, but it must be in context. Some people read or are told about the side effects of medications (or other treatments) and say, "Wow, look at the risks! I'm not going to do that!" But not doing something may also have risks. Not taking a treatment may mean that the illness will get worse or more complicated. The potential benefits and risks of any decision should be carefully considered by you and your doctor.

It's also important to be aware that there are generic side effects that have nothing to do with particular medications. For example, many tablets contain lactose, and this may affect those people with extreme lactose intolerance. Some tablets are large and difficult to swallow. Various medications used in IBD are taken in the form of an enema; there is a small but real risk of puncturing the rectum with the plastic enema tip. Suppositories can irritate the anal canal.

Drug Interactions

Interactions can make a drug less effective or can change a usual dose into an overdose or an underdose. Any time a new drug is given to you, make sure that the prescriber knows all the other drugs that you take, whether daily or intermittent, and whether prescribed or over-the-counter. Also ask your pharmacist to check for possible interactions; to make this check most effective, it's a good idea to get all your drugs at the same pharmacy (or at least at the same chain, provided there's a shared database).

And it's not just drugs that can potentially interact. For example, the phytochemicals curcumin (found in the spice turmeric) and catechins (found in green tea) inhibit the therapeutic effects of anti-TNF drugs (see page 85).

Biological Therapy

The term "biologicals" (sometimes "biologics") has been coined to describe a powerful class of drugs that has arisen as a result of the science of molecular biology, and our ability to use this science to develop new therapies. The approval of this form of treatment in 1998 in the United States and Canada, among other countries, was a milestone in IBD management. Until then, unless there was an urgent situation, IBD therapy typically followed a "step-up" approach, beginning with the least potent drugs (which generally have the fewest and least serious side effects) and progressing gradually "up the ladder" to more and more potent drugs. Since the arrival of biologicals on the scene, there has been much discussion about using a "step-down" approach to therapy. The idea is to begin with our most powerful drugs to rapidly bring the disease under control, and to then consider gradually going "down the ladder" to less powerful drugs to try to keep the disease controlled. However, the majority of doctors in the field agree that the most practical approach is one of an *individualized strategy* now called "personalized" medicine. We should consider that every patient is different and requires a thoughtful, personalized approach. Some people will need the most potent therapy right away, while others will never need it. The treatment should match the severity of the disease.

Combination Therapy

Generally, physicians in the field believe that most classes of drugs used to treat IBD work in different ways. The result of this is that we frequently use combinations of drugs. Unfortunately, very few combinations have been studied in a meaningful way. Most patients end up on combination therapy because they are not doing well, and their doctors are trying to make them better. The downside for patients is that they end up taking more medication without knowing whether it is worthwhile or not.

Drugs used to treat IBD can be divided into two categories. The first includes those that reduce inflammation, and in turn reducing symptoms such as diarrhea and pain. The second includes those that have no effect on inflammation but may be useful in reducing or eliminating symptoms, especially diarrhea and crampy pain. In both categories, I discuss only some of the side effects (a full discussion is beyond the scope of this book). Of course, in addition to drugs there are several nondrug therapies, such as dietary changes, covered in Chapter 5, and surgery, which is covered in Chapter 7.

Drugs That Reduce Inflammation
Sulfasalazine
In the late 1930s, Dr. Nana Svartz, a Swedish researcher, proposed linking one of the newly discovered sulfa drugs with acetylsalicylic acid (i.e., Aspirin or ASA), to treat the painful joint disease rheumatoid arthritis, at that time thought to be caused by an infection. The first patient Dr. Svartz treated with such a combined drug, called sulfasalazine, happened to have ulcerative colitis as well. The most striking benefit for this patient was control of his colitis. Until the introduction of sulfasalazine in 1942, no medication had been able to control colitis. For the next 8 years it remained the only drug available for the treatment of colitis — until cortisone was introduced in 1950. Sulfasalazine continued to be the only drug in its class until the 1980s, when pure 5-ASA (5-aminosalicylate, the active ingredient of sulfasalazine) became available.

Most gastroenterologists now prefer to prescribe the pure 5-ASA drugs, but some still start with sulfasalazine, particularly if the patient also has arthritis. Pure 5-ASA does not have any value in arthritis, whereas sulfasalazine does for some patients. Compared with pure 5-ASA, sulfasalazine is just as effective, and it's cheaper. But sulfasalazine has side effects much more often than pure 5-ASA.

Sulfasalazine comes in tablets, either coated or uncoated.

How Does It Work?
The 5-aminosalicylate (5-ASA) portion of sulfasalazine limits the production of certain chemical products of inflammation that promote diarrhea. It also removes oxygen radicals from tissues. These substances, released during inflammation, are toxic to cells. Like all sulfa drugs, sulfasalazine is an antibacterial agent. This means that it prevents some bacteria from functioning and causing illness, though it does not kill them. The antibacterial activity is not thought to be important in ulcerative colitis. It may have some value in Crohn's disease, but there is not much evidence for this, even though some antibiotics — which kill bacteria — are clearly beneficial.

When Is It Used?

Sulfasalazine can be used to treat mild to moderate attacks of ulcerative colitis and Crohn's disease. But it is most valuable because it reduces the chance of a flare-up of ulcerative colitis, and probably Crohn's colitis as well, in many people. If taken regularly, it continues to have this effect indefinitely. A similar effect has not been proven in small bowel Crohn's disease, but some people with Crohn's in that location appear to do well on the drug. Sulfasalazine may also be used to treat arthritis, which occurs in about 20 percent of people with IBD.

What Are the Side Effects?

The most frequent side effects of sulfasalazine are gastrointestinal. Nausea and reduced appetite are common, but of course these can also be symptoms of IBD. Vomiting is less common. These side effects can sometimes be prevented if you start with a small dose of the drug and increase it slowly, rather than starting with a full dose on the first day. It also helps to take the pills with food rather than on an empty stomach. A coated form of sulfasalazine releases the drug more slowly and is particularly helpful in reducing nausea due to the drug.

The second most common type of side effect is an allergic reaction. This usually appears as an itchy rash (hives) or swelling of the hands or face, or both. In someone who has never taken sulfasalazine before, the reaction generally occurs 14 to 21 days after starting the drug. In someone who has taken the drug before, it generally occurs within the first week. Report any allergic reactions to your doctor immediately. About 70 percent of the people who have an allergic reaction can be desensitized, so that the drug can be gradually reintroduced. Occasionally, allergic reactions will be associated with arthritis (inflamed joints), hepatitis (inflamed liver), fever or many other inflammations of tissues and organs. Desensitization should not be attempted in such cases.

The third type of common side effect involves the blood. Red blood cells normally have a life span of 120 days. These blood cells are then taken up by the spleen, destroyed, and replaced by new red blood cells from the bone marrow, in a normal process that goes on all the time. In some people, sulfasalazine causes the red blood cells to be destroyed prematurely. This process is called hemolysis, from "heme," meaning blood, and "lysis," meaning breakdown. Hemolysis is generally reversible and can be controlled in some patients simply by reducing the dose of sulfasalazine; in others, the drug must be stopped completely.

Another blood-related side effect of sulfasalazine is that it can reduce the ability of the intestine to absorb folic acid, possibly leading to anemia. Folic acid (known as folate when it occurs naturally in foods), is one of the B vitamins and one of the building blocks of red blood cells. Physicians will prescribe a daily folic acid pill when necessary.

A very rare but serious side effect of sulfasalazine is bone-marrow shutdown (marrow aplasia). In addition to red blood cells, the bone marrow makes white blood cells and platelets. With this side effect, the production of any or all types of blood cells may stop. Treatments for this exist but are not always effective, and death can result. Bone-marrow shutdown usually occurs within the first three months of therapy, but it also represents the most serious long-term risk of sulfasalazine. Unusual bleeding or bruising should be reported immediately to your doctor.

Up to 80 percent of men taking sulfasalazine will have a reduced sperm count enough to make them infertile. In addition, the sperm are less active and may have an abnormal appearance. Stopping the drug allows the count to return to normal, though this may take up to two months. This side effect does not occur with pure 5-ASA.

Headaches can also occur with sulfasalazine. In some people they are mild, but in others they are severe enough that the drug must be stopped. Many patients who take sulfasalazine notice that their urine is orange-yellow. Yellowing of the skin and of soft contact lenses has occasionally been reported, but this discoloration is harmless.

In rare cases, an attack of ulcerative colitis, or a worsening of an attack, will occur with sulfasalazine. The drug must be stopped and the attack treated in some other way.

Pure 5-Aminosalicylate (5-ASA)
The active ingredient in sulfasalazine, 5-aminosalicylate (5-ASA), does not have any antibacterial properties. Although it is chemically similar to ASA, 5-ASA doesn't do anything that ASA does, and ASA doesn't do anything that 5-ASA does.

How Does It Work?
Like sulfasalazine, 5-ASA reduces the production of diarrhea-causing chemicals in the intestine. It also inactivates oxygen radicals that destroy tissue.

When Is It Used?

5-ASA can be used to treat mild to moderate attacks of ulcerative colitis and Crohn's disease. For people with proctitis or colitis limited to the last 1 to 2 feet (30 to 60 centimeters) of the colon, small doses taken rectally can be more effective than much larger doses taken orally. For many people, the greatest value of this drug is that it reduces the chance of flare-ups of both ulcerative colitis and Crohn's colitis; it can also provide this benefit in some people with small bowel Crohn's disease. Used postoperatively, 5-ASA has been shown, in some studies, to reduce the risk of recurrent small bowel Crohn's disease (only in patients with isolated small bowel Crohn's disease prior to surgery), though the reduction is modest at best and this benefit is lost if the patient smokes.

Common Questions About 5-ASA

Q: Is one 5-ASA product better than any other for the treatment of small bowel Crohn's disease?

A: The 5-ASA products that target the small bowel and colon are all approximately equal; the minor differences in formulation have not been studied comparatively.

Q: Is there any evidence that a person with colitis should be treated with a 5-ASA product that is targeted specifically at the colon?

A: While there are some published data suggesting that this is the case, the evidence is not compelling. It appears that all the oral forms are effective in colitis.

Q: Is there any point in trying 5-ASA enemas or suppositories if oral 5-ASA does not appear to be working?

A: Definitely yes. Rectally administered 5-ASA is often effective (even in very small doses) when oral 5-ASA is not (even in maximum doses).

Q: If I am doing well on sulfasalazine, should I switch to a pure 5-ASA product?

A: Most gastroenterologists agree that you should not switch. There is a somewhat greater risk of diarrhea as a side effect with 5-ASA; this is unpredictable and occasionally severe.

Q: If my ulcerative colitis has been inactive for several years, should I stop my sulfasalazine or 5-ASA medication?

A: Not without asking your doctor first. The main function of these medications is to reduce the risk of flare-up. There may also be a cancer prevention benefit.

What Are the Side Effects?
Many of the side effects of 5-ASA are similar to those of sulfasalazine. But they occur much less commonly, because the sulfa portion of sulfasalazine is responsible for many of those adverse effects is absent in 5-ASA.

The main side effects include nausea and headaches. Diarrhea occurs occasionally — more with one form of the drug, olsalazine, than with others. The diarrhea may be reduced by introducing the drug gradually and taking it with food.

Other less common side effects include allergic reactions (e.g., itchy rash and swelling of the hands and face, fever). As with sulfasalazine, some allergic patients can be desensitized. A severe, dull, steady pain across the upper abdomen, sometimes with back pain, may indicate pancreatitis (inflammation of the pancreas). If pancreatitis occurs, 5-ASA cannot be used again. This drug has no effect on sperm count or fertility.

As with sulfasalazine, in rare cases an attack of ulcerative colitis or a worsening of an attack will occur with 5-ASA. The drug must be stopped and the attack treated in some other way.

Hair loss has occasionally been reported as a side effect, but the reliability of the reports is questionable. There is a normal process of hair turnover, in which a certain number of hairs fall out every day and are replaced by new ones. It is extremely common for this turnover to be accelerated during an illness, and especially in the weeks afterward; the name for this is telogen effluvium. You may notice more hair in your comb or brush, and more hair in the shower or bathtub drain. If you have long hair, you are much more likely to notice that your hair looks or feels thinner, as the new hair coming in is short. The observation of this type of hair loss almost always comes from women, and they often have to temporarily change hair style. But the loss is temporary; new hair is growing in. Hair loss is serious only if the hair comes out in clumps and leaves bald patches. This type of hair loss has been reported with 5-ASA only very rarely.

Because brands of drugs come and go, in this book I have used generic drug names. For the brand-name drugs available in 2011, see Appendix I on page 216.

Patients commonly use 5-ASA enemas or suppositories as maintenance therapy. The chronic use of any sort of enema or suppository can irritate the anal canal and produce pain and bleeding.

Kidney damage is a very rare side effect of 5-ASA. It is not unusual for patients on this drug to have an excessive number of white blood cells in their urine. Having your urine and kidney function checked periodically (e.g., once yearly) when you use 5-ASA is recommended. 5-ASA is available in tablet, enema and suppository form. A rectal foam is on the market in some countries but not in North America.

Several brands of 5-ASA tablets are available. Each brand "targets" the 5-ASA to specific sites in the intestine. Whether these differences are of clinical significance has not yet been demonstrated. Newer formulations, as well as some of the older products, can be taken once or twice a day, rather than three to four times a day, as in the past.

Generic names for 5-ASA products include mesalamine, mesalazine and olsalazine. The newest product in this group is balsalazide, which consists of a unit of 5-ASA linked to an inert carrier. Research suggests that balsalazide may be a little more effective than the pure 5-ASA products, but more studies are needed.

Steroids
Glucocorticoids (or glucocorticosteroids), the steroids used to treat IBD, are derivatives of cortisol, a natural steroid produced by the adrenal glands, which sit on top of the kidneys. Glucocorticoids are different from the anabolic steroids used by some athletes to enhance performance. The first glucocorticoid to be given to patients was cortisone, in 1950. The introduction of this potent drug revolutionized the treatment of many chronic diseases, including IBD. Currently, the most-used glucocorticoids are prednisone and prednisolone.

How Do They Work?
Quite simply, glucocorticoids reduce inflammation. The details of this are beyond the scope of this book, but you'll find plenty of information online, as well as in bookstores.

When Are They Used?
Steroids are used to treat many moderate and severe attacks of ulcerative colitis and Crohn's disease. In people with ulcerative colitis,

once the attack has settled down significantly, the dose should gradually be reduced to zero over several weeks. There is no evidence that steroids prevent flare-ups of ulcerative colitis, so people with this disease should generally not remain on this medication between attacks. However, about 5 percent of ulcerative colitis patients have what is referred to as chronic continuous colitis, and with these people, it may not be possible to get the steroid dosage down to zero between attacks, Many of these patients require continuous therapy to stay well, unless an effective alternative is used.

It is much more common for people to require continuous steroid therapy in Crohn's disease than in ulcerative colitis, to suppress chronic symptoms. In such cases, it is usually desirable to try to switch to "steroid-sparing" therapies, such as immunosuppressives or biologicals, or both. Some people are said to be "steroid-dependent"; this means that they either can't get off steroids or that they need frequent steroids. Some people need to avoid steroids because of intolerable side effects. The aim of steroid-sparing therapy is to eliminate steroid dependency or, in some cases, to allow the patient to require only very low doses of steroids. Nevertheless, many people with Crohn's disease require steroids only intermittently. Still others do not need them at all. Steroids do not prevent Crohn's disease from recurring after surgery.

If you need long-term steroid therapy, your doctor may tell you to try taking a double dose every second day and skipping the days in between — known as alternate-day dosing. It is supposed to be just as effective, with fewer net side effects. However, many people complain that they simply do not feel as well on the off days, so this dosing is not widely used.

When either ulcerative colitis or Crohn's colitis is limited to the last 1 to 2 feet (30 to 60 centimeters) of the colon, steroids may be just as effective rectally as similar or larger doses taken orally, with far fewer side effects.

What Are the Side Effects?
Steroids have both visible and invisible side effects.
Visible side effects. Although these may be upsetting to you, they *are* reversible weeks to months after the drug has been stopped, with the possible exception of excessive weight gain. Also, these side effects are not dangerous in themselves. They include:
• rounding of the face — appears gradually;

- redness of the face, usually mild — creates a "healthier" appearance;
- increased appetite and weight gain, often desirable;
- mood changes — often happier because of feeling better; feeling nervous or jittery; being irritable; serious extremes of mood such as euphoria or severe depression are very uncommon;
- acne — mild to severe; may require antibiotics; mostly in individuals taking steroids for weeks or more; usually improves with dose reduction but occasionally first appears, or becomes much worse, shortly after steroids stopped;
- increased energy and insomnia — some people sleep fewer hours and yet do not get sleepy during the day; you may need a sleeping pill temporarily, particularly with big doses;
- ankle swelling in malnourished people;
- weakness of the muscles of the thighs and upper arms; difficulty climbing stairs and getting up from a seat without using your arms;
- night sweats — may also be a sign of illness;
- facial hair growth — rarely noticeable, but very annoying to some women;
- skinny arms, a pot belly and, in some people, a hump of fat on the middle of the upper back — with long-term therapy (i.e., years);
- easy bruising and thinning of the skin; mainly with long-term therapy (i.e., years);
- possibly reduced growth rate and delayed puberty (see Chapter 8);
- muscle and joint stiffness soon after a course of oral steroids is completed.

Invisible side effects. These are of greater concern because they can cause irreversible harm:
- softening of the bones (osteoporosis) — especially hips and spine; mainly with long-term therapy (i.e., years); physical inactivity, malnutrition, vitamin D deficiency and a low-lactose diet increase risk, which can be monitored with bone densitometry (bone-density testing);
- death of a portion of bone (osteonecrosis, also known as avascular necrosis) — especially hips and knees; even with short-term therapy (i.e., weeks); this rare side effect can also occur in IBD without steroids; treatment is usually by artificial joint replacement;
- reduced immunity — increased risk of infections; mainly with high

doses, hospitalized patients and combination therapy with other drugs that suppress the immune system; it's important to remember that severe illness and malnutrition also suppress the immune system, so effective treatment of the IBD improves immune function;

- aggravation of diabetes mellitus — increased blood sugar, usually temporary;
- cataracts — mainly with higher doses and prolonged therapy;
- increased eye pressure (glaucoma) — more common in children;
- reduced potassium level, also a result of diarrhea; can contribute to weakness;
- high blood pressure — very uncommon;
- ulcers of the stomach or duodenum, or both (controversial); only with high doses, if at all.

FORMS OF STEROIDS

There are many forms of cortisone-like steroids. They are available as tablets (e.g., prednisone, prednisolone), injectable forms (e.g., hydrocortisone, methylprednisolone), suppositories (e.g., hydrocortisone), enemas and rectal foams.

People being treated with rectal steroids can often retain suppositories or foam much more easily than liquid enemas, sometimes with equal benefit. Most rectal steroids are only partially absorbed into the bloodstream, so that side effects are minimized. This is particularly true for hydrocortisone-containing products.

Budesonide is a newer steroid, available as oral capsules and as an enema. It has fewer short-term side effects; this is thought to be because it acts locally, at the site of disease in the intestine. However, we know that oral budesonide can be effective in left-sided colitis; since it is supposed to be absorbed in the ileum, it is clear that that there is a systemic effect as well. When budesonide is absorbed into the bloodstream, it is metabolized (broken down) rapidly into components with low steroid activity. If a patient has chronic liver disease, the metabolism of budesonide may be impaired, resulting in a greater systemic effect. With long-term use of budesonide, the kinds of side effects listed above may appear, though there is some evidence that osteoporosis may be less of a problem. If a person is being switched from one of the other oral steroids (e.g., prednisone) to budesonide, symptoms of adrenal insufficiency (see Stopping Steroids on page 80) may occur.

Important Points to Remember About Steroid Therapy
- Never stop steroids suddenly unless clearly advised to do so by your doctor. The usual practice is to taper the dose until it is down to zero, although if steroids have been taken for 2 weeks or less, they *can* be stopped abruptly if this is desired.
- Always advise *any* physician, dentist or paramedical person treating you that you are or have been on steroids within the previous 12 months. Some physicians recommend that you wear a medical-alert bracelet or necklace if you're on steroids.
- Remind your physician that you have been on steroids within the previous 12 months if you are being treated with an acute illness. Your doctor must keep track of hundreds of patients; you have only one — you.

STOPPING STEROIDS

The last of the invisible side effects (see page 79) may occur days to months after you stop taking steroids. As mentioned earlier, your body normally makes cortisol (a steroid similar to prednisone or prednisolone) in the adrenal glands, little glands that sit on the top of the kidneys. When your body is subjected to physical stress (e.g., fever, surgery), it produces up to 10 times more cortisol than under normal conditions. With extreme psychological stress, there can be a very temporary increase in cortisol. When you take steroids, normal cortisol production decreases or stops completely. When you stop taking the steroid, production begins again but may be sluggish for up to a year. This means that you may need to take steroids at a time of physical stress, for up to 12 months after you have come off the medication. The steroids may be necessary for days or longer, depending on the illness. If the stress is mental, and extreme, the steroids should be taken for only 1 to 2 days, if at all. *Any use of steroids in these circumstances should be discussed first with your doctor.*

Symptoms of insufficient cortisol (the technical term is adrenal insufficiency) are nonspecific. They include nausea, extreme fatigue, weakness, light-headedness and possibly diarrhea. If your body goes without adequate steroids long enough, the condition can be fatal. If you suspect that you are not producing enough cortisol soon after stopping steroids, discuss it with your doctor.

Immunosuppressive (Immunomodulator) Drugs

Immunosuppressives are another class of drugs used in the treatment of IBD. They were originally introduced to treat certain cancers. They have also been used to help prevent rejection in organ transplants. In both these situations, relatively large doses of the drugs are administered. It has been known for more than 55 years, however, that smaller doses of immunosuppressives can be used effectively to treat various other conditions, including IBD. The most exciting recent development with this class of drugs has been the demonstration that some of them can heal Crohn's disease. But remember, healing is not curing. If something is cured, treatment can be stopped. Doctors believe that to maintain healing, treatment should continue.

How Do They Work?

Different drugs in this class work in different ways. The desired result is to rebalance the immune system (see Chapter 2). Eventually, the term immunomodulator (meaning modifying immune function) will probably replace the term immunosuppressive, reflecting the expansion of this class of drugs.

When Are They Used?

These drugs are most often used when there is a desire to reduce, eliminate or avoid the use of steroids. Both ulcerative colitis patients and Crohn's disease patients who need frequent or continuous steroid therapy can often reduce their dosage, or get off steroids altogether. Once disease control has been achieved, many people stay well for years, and studies have confirmed that this long-lasting benefit is real. Some of these drugs are also used to try and prevent Crohn's disease from coming back after surgery. In ulcerative colitis, immunosuppressive drugs usually work within 2 to 12 weeks, if there is going to be a response. Because these drugs tend to act more slowly in Crohn's disease, you may have to wait up to 6 months or more for a benefit. Because the drugs act so slowly, it is often necessary to increase steroids temporarily.

Here is a typical case. A 27-year-old man with Crohn's disease sought a second opinion because he could not stop taking prednisone. He had a history of extensive surgery, so another operation was undesirable.

Despite prednisone, he was having daily crampy pain and diarrhea. He was put on azathioprine. One month later he was told to try to reduce the prednisone. He promptly began to have more symptoms of Crohn's disease and had to increase the prednisone again. One month later, he again reduced the prednisone, with the same result. The next month all of his Crohn's symptoms gradually disappeared. He was then able to gradually reduce and then stop the prednisone. He continued on the azathioprine alone and remained well.

What Are the Side Effects?
Larger doses of immunosuppressives — such as those used in transplant patients and people being treated for certain types of cancer — increase the risk of malignancy, particularly lymphoma. Although there has been controversy about this in the past, recent studies have shown that there is an increased risk of lymphoma, compared with the general population, with azathioprine and 6-mercaptopurine, even with the lower doses used in IBD. We don't have enough data to say whether this occurs with methotrexate, although we know that this drug does increase the lymphoma risk in other conditions.

All immunosuppressive drugs reduce the effectiveness of your immune system, though this is relatively mild with the doses used for IBD. Resistance to infections decreases, and this can be serious in the case of unusual infections that may be difficult to diagnose and treat. You should report any fever, chills or persistent sore throat to your doctor promptly. In some types of infection, your doctor may tell you to temporarily stop your immunosuppressive.

Side effects of specific drugs are listed below.

The Main Immunosuppressive Drugs
The main immunosuppressive drugs used are as follows:

AZATHIOPRINE AND 6-MERCAPTOPURINE
- Used in IBD for more than 55 years.
- An excellent long-term strategy for many people with IBD.
- Azathioprine and 6-mercaptopurine are equally effective.
- Convenient once-a-day dose.
- Can heal (not cure) both Crohn's disease and ulcerative colitis in some people.

- Side effects occur in about 15 percent of people.
- Some side effects (nausea, rash) with one may not occur with the other.
- Liver inflammation (hepatitis) can occur early or later on.
- Lowering of blood cell counts is reversible but occasionally life-threatening.
- Lowering of white blood cell count is enhanced by all 5-ASA drugs.
- Pancreatitis can occur weeks or months after starting.
- Increased risk of skin cancer.
- Slight increased risk of lymphoma compared with the general population (see the Risk of Serious Events table, page 92), but either a decreased risk, or no effect on risk, of all other types of cancer (except for skin cancer, as noted above).

METHOTREXATE
- Available for 60 years, but first used in IBD in the late 1980s.
- Often given by injection, but sometimes effective by mouth.
- Once-weekly dosing is attractive.
- You must also take folic acid (folate, a B vitamin) — the dose is controversial, so check with your doctor.
- A good alternative to azathioprine or 6-mercaptopurine for Crohn's disease — may be effective in ulcerative colitis, but evidence is weak so far.
- Benefit is expected within 2 to 12 weeks of starting therapy.
- Common side effects are nausea and mouth ulcers, reduced by folate supplementation.
- Bone marrow suppression much less than with azathioprine or 6-mercaptopurine.
- Can rarely cause cirrhosis of the liver with long-term use; risk increased in the presence of alcohol use, obesity and diabetes.

CYCLOSPORINE (CYCLOSPORIN A)
- First used for IBD in the late 1980s.
- Has potentially severe side effects, including kidney damage, high blood pressure and liver damage, when used long term.
- Causes increased facial hair and enlargement of the gums.
- Risk of side effects reduced by monitoring drug blood levels.
- Main use is to reduce need for urgent surgery in severe ulcerative coli-

tis, but many of those people still need surgery within 6 to 12 months.
- Usually replaced by azathioprine, 6-mercaptopurine or a biological if attack subsides.
- Available in oral or intravenous forms.

TACROLIMUS
- An antibiotic with immunosuppressive properties.
- First used as an antirejection drug in transplantation.
- Studied for IBD since 1995.
- Used occasionally, mainly in IBD centers.
- Common side effects include tremor, elevated blood sugar, high blood pressure, kidney damage and infection — none is considered severe.
- Available as a cream for Crohn's perianal disease and for pyoderma gangrenosum (see Chapter 9).

MYCOPHENOLATE MOFETIL (MMF)
- First used as an anti-rejection drug in transplantation.
- Studied for IBD since 1998.
- Used occasionally, mainly in IBD centers.
- Common side effects include nausea.
- Can cause a drug-induced colitis *but* has been used with success in both Crohn's colitis and ulcerative colitis, as well as small bowel Crohn's disease.

THALIDOMIDE, LENALIDOMIDE
- Thalidomide is an old drug for nausea due to pregnancy — caused serious birth defects.
- Has anti-TNF activity (see discussion of infliximab on page 85).
- Studied in both ulcerative colitis and Crohn's disease.
- Common side effects include mild drowsiness, dry mouth, dry skin, and tingling, burning, numbness or pain in the hands, arms, feet or legs.
- Lenalidomide is a newer (but similar) drug than thalidomide.
- Most doctors agree that more study of both agents is needed.

Biologicals (Biologics)

The term "biologicals" has been coined to describe a powerful class of drugs that has arisen as a result of the science of molecular biology, and our ability to use this science to develop new therapies. The main characteristic of these agents is that they target specific molecules involved in the inflammatory process. The best-known biologicals are in the anti-TNF family. At the time of writing, several anti-TNF biologicals are approved for use in some countries for the treatment of IBD, ankylosing spondylitis (a form of arthritis that occurs mainly in people with IBD), rheumatoid arthritis, psoriasis, some other autoimmune diseases and asthma. These include infliximab, adalimumab, certolizumab pegol, golimumab and ustekinemab. Natalizumab is another approved biological, with a different mechanism of action. Visilizumab is another anti-TNF drug, in an advanced state of development but not yet on the market.

Anti-TNFs

INFLIXIMAB

This drug was the first of the biologicals. Infliximab is a murine, chimeric, monoclonal antibody directed toward tumor necrosis factor–alpha (TNF-alpha). "Murine" means that it's produced in mice; "chimeric" means that its chemistry is a blend of two species — it's about 75 percent human protein and 25 percent mouse protein. Because it's directed at TNF-alpha it is often referred to as an anti-TNF drug.

Don't be alarmed. This treatment has nothing to do with tumors; the name relates to the way TNF was discovered. The word necrosis means cell destruction, but this treatment does not destroy cells. Infliximab is given by intravenous infusion. People with Crohn's disease or ulcerative colitis are given an initial course of three infusions, referred to as an induction dose or "loading dose"; the second infusion is 2 weeks after the first, and the third is 4 weeks after that. The usual maintenance schedule is one infusion every 8 weeks, beginning 8 weeks after the third loading dose. If infliximab is effective, but the effect isn't lasting the full 8 weeks, the interval between infusions can be shortened, most typically to every 6 weeks. If there is no response to the drug, or if response has occurred and then is lost, doubling the dose is sometimes effective.

The main disadvantages of infliximab are that you need to go to an outpatient clinic to receive it, and the IV infusion takes 1 to 2 hours. However, despite the inconvenience, this drug was the first on the market in this class and has been used extensively. At the time of writing, it has been given to close to 1.5 million people, mainly people with IBD or rheumatoid arthritis. To date, it is the best studied in its class and has the best published results.

ADALIMUMAB

This anti-TNF agent is referred to as a humanized monoclonal antibody, which means it doesn't contain any mouse protein. It is given as a subcutaneous injection, which means it's injected into the fat just under the skin. The standard induction protocol (loading dose) is 160 milligrams (mg) (four injections) the first time, 80 mg (two injections) 2 weeks later, and 40 mg (one injection) 2 weeks after that. Most people will then receive one injection of 40 mg every 2 weeks thereafter. If adalimumab is effective but the effect isn't lasting the full 2 weeks, the interval between injections can be shortened, most typically to every week. If there is no response to the drug, changing the schedule to weekly injections is sometimes useful.

The main advantages of adalimumab over infliximab are that most patients give it to themselves at home, and it takes just a few seconds. Most patients just need one tutorial to learn to do this. But not all patients are comfortable giving themselves injections, and some people develop a needle phobia after a period of time. Adalimumab is currently marketed in two forms: the self-injection pen, and a preloaded syringe, more likely to be used if someone is giving you the injection. Next to infliximab, this drug has had the most study. At the time of writing, it has been given to more than half a million people. Its published results in IBD are not quite as good as infliximab but certainly respectable.

CERTOLIZUMAB PEGOL

This anti-TNF drug is yet another variation on the monoclonal antibody model. It too doesn't have any mouse protein. This anti-TNF agent is also given as a subcutaneous injection. The standard induction protocol (loading dose) is 400 milligrams (mg) the first time, 400 mg 2 weeks later, 400 mg another 2 weeks later, and then 400 mg once a month. At the time of writing, the drug must be prepared just before use. It can be taken as a self-injection (again, one tutorial on how to do this is usually enough) or can be given to you by a nurse or doctor. The manufacturer is working on a self-injection pen. At the time of writing, this drug is on the market for the treatment of Crohn's disease only in the United States and Switzerland. However, it is on the market in both the United States and Canada for the treatment of rheumatoid arthritis.

GOLIMUMAB

This anti-TNF agent has been approved for use in the treatment of ankylosing spondylitis, rheumatoid arthritis and psoriatic arthritis, and may be approved for IBD in the near future.

ETANERCEPT

Another anti-TNF antibody, etanercept, is 100 percent human. It is used for several kinds of arthritis, including ankylosing spondylitis (see Chapter 9). Studies in IBD have been disappointing, which is frustrating for those IBD patients who also have ankylosing spondylitis and are doing well on etanercept but need a change in therapy for their IBD.

Main Benefits and Drawbacks of Anti-TNFs

Two of the great benefits of anti-TNF drugs are that they work quickly (for infliximab, within 2 weeks, and sometimes as fast as 24 hours) and that they can heal (not cure) Crohn's disease and ulcerative colitis. The biggest drawback of these drugs (and all biologicals) is cost. Because dosing of infliximab is based on the patient's body weight, there is some variation in the cost, but the average annual cost is in the range of $40,000 to $60,000. Adalimumab dosing is the same for all patients; the only variation after the induction doses is that some people receive a weekly dose, though most take it every 2 weeks. This standardizes the cost, but it is similar to infliximab on an annual basis. Clearly this kind of expense is beyond the reach of all but the very rich, so private insurance or government support, or some combination, is essential.

How Do They Work?

TNF is a major promoter of inflammation. It also has an important function in keeping certain dormant diseases in check. In simple terms, anti-TNF drugs work by blocking the effects of TNF. Many of the details of how this is achieved are still to be worked out.

How Long Does the Benefit of These Drugs Last?
The duration of the benefit is quite variable. It averages 6 to 8 weeks for infliximab. If the benefit starts to wear off before the 8-week mark, then the interval between infusions is shortened, usually to every 6 or 7 weeks. Some patients feel they need the drug even more frequently than every 6 weeks; unfortunately, many funding agencies (governments, insurance companies) refuse to pay for the shorter intervals. For ulcerative colitis, some funding agencies will pay for this drug only every 8 weeks and require evidence of continuing benefit at regular intervals (usually a few months).

If an IBD patient on adalimumab reports reduction or loss of benefit before the 2-week mark, the injections can be given as frequently as every 7 days.

When Are They Used?
At the time of writing, the main reasons to use these medications in IBD is for people with moderate or severe Crohn's disease or ulcerative colitis that is unresponsive or poorly responsive to other conventional therapies. Early evidence suggests they may also reduce the risk of Crohn's disease coming back after surgery. For many years, the conventional approach to treating IBD has been to start with the least potent drugs (which often have few serious side effects) and progress step by step to the most potent drugs. This is known as the step-up approach. More recently, some doctors have favored beginning with the most potent therapy (to theoretically have the best chance of controlling the disease), with the idea of then stepping down to less potent medication to maintain remission. This is known as the step-down approach. However, as discussed at the beginning of this chapter, more than ever, doctors are trying to match patients' treatments to their problem at the time. Anti-TNF therapies can be particularly helpful for Crohn's patients with complex fistulas but, like every treatment for Crohn's disease, it works only in some people. These drugs are much more likely to work in nonsmokers. It appears too that they sometimes work better in people who are also on immunosuppressives.

Anti-TNF drugs are also used in people with some of the other manifestations of IBD, such as ankylosing spondylitis and pyoderma gangrenosum (see Chapter 9).

So far, the only other common diseases being treated with this class of drug are rheumatoid arthritis and psoriasis.

Is it worthwhile to try a second anti-TNF if you haven't responded to the first one? Yes, definitely, although the chance of response is lower than the chance of response in someone being treated for the first time.

What Are the Side Effects?

The monitoring of drug safety in general has been facilitated by the widespread use of computer databases. An excellent example of this is the Crohn's disease Therapy, Evaluation and Assessment Tool (TREAT) registry. This large database of Crohn's disease patients was created specifically to document adverse effects to the first anti-TNF drug, infliximab. In the United States, the Food and Drug Administration has an adverse-event reporting system that can be accessed by the public through the MedWatch portal; although this has some significant drawbacks, it is another source of information.

Although reading the list of side effects of these drugs can be scary, the fact is that most people do not experience any side effects. In Crohn's disease studies, about 5 percent of patients had to stop receiving the drug because of side effects. The main reasons were infusion (intravenous) reactions (this applies to infliximab only), local skin

---

Tell Your Doctor

Before starting anti-TNF therapy, inform your doctor if you have, or ever had:

- tuberculosis (TB) or if you have been near someone who has TB;
- lived in a region where certain fungal infections such as histoplasmosis or coccidioidomycosis are common;
- infections that keep coming back, have diabetes or an immune system problem;
- heart failure or any heart condition — many people with heart failure should not take anti-TNF drugs;
- hepatitis B virus (HBV), or hepatitis C virus (HCV), or HIV-AIDS infection, or think you may be a carrier of HBV, HCV or HIV;
- nervous system disorders (such as MS or previous Guillain-Barré syndrome);
- if you have never had chicken pox.

reactions (adalimumab or certolizumab injections) or subsequent infections. Typical reactions include headache, nausea, light-headedness, flushing and hives. A few people develop chest pain or shortness of breath. Infusion reactions to infliximab are fairly common, occurring in about 15 percent of people, but most are mild and do not require the drug to be withdrawn. In less than 1 percent of cases does the infusion have to be stopped and not restarted; usually it can be restarted at a slower rate, or after administration of a medication such as an antihistamine, or acetaminophen for headache.

Another side effect is an increased risk of infection, especially tuberculosis and fungal infections. Some of these infections are serious, and some are life-threatening. Many people carry dormant tuberculosis (TB) bacteria, and an important beneficial function of TNF is preventing the TB from becoming active. In some people, when the TNF is blocked, active TB infection occurs. This seems to happen mostly to people who are on additional immunosuppressive medications. This has led to the standard practice of having anyone who is going to be treated to first have a TB skin test and a chest X-ray. If there is evidence of TB, it must be treated first, or anti-TNF therapy should not be given. Other, and sometimes unusual, infections may also occur as a result of anti-TNF therapy. Some physicians now routinely test for immunity to varicella virus (chicken pox) and hepatitis A, B and C, and advise vaccination for chicken pox and hepatitis A and B if the patient is not already immune. There is no vaccine as yet for hepatitis C, but knowing that someone is a carrier allows better monitoring. At the time of writing, advance testing for HIV is controversial; so far, reports have not indicated a particular problem in HIV-positive individuals. Despite the fact that anti-TNFs are sometimes used to treat chronic skin diseases, the first appearance of psoriasis and other chronic skin conditions has been reported to be a newly recognized side effect.

ANTIBODY FORMATION WITH ANTI-TNF THERAPY
Some people taking anti-TNF drugs develop antinuclear antibodies (ANA, also known as ANF, for "antinuclear factor"). These antibodies are frequently present in people with the disease known as lupus (systemic lupus erythematosus, or SLE). Some people (with or without IBD) test positive for lupus without having the disease. A few people treated with anti-TNFs and who have a positive ANA test will

later develop lupus, which will likely require treatment with steroids. Several drugs used to treat other conditions are also known to cause lupus or a lupus-like condition.

Two other types of antibodies occur with anti-TNFs. Some people develop antibodies to the specific anti-TNF drug they are taking. This sounds like a bad thing, but many people with such antibodies maintain their response to the treatment. It has been shown that simultaneous treatment with immunosuppressives reduces such antibody formation, but whether this is really necessary is controversial.

A second type of antibody, HACA (human anti-chimeric antibody), is specific to infliximab and correlates with infusion reactions. Having these antibodies can reduce the effectiveness of the drug. If you have responded to infliximab and then have lost your response, measurement of drug levels may be useful. If levels are low, an increased dose of infliximab may allow you to regain your response. If your blood drug levels are not low, then the preferred strategy is to switch to a different anti-TNF. It has been shown that simultaneous treatment with immunosuppressives, even in low doses, also reduces this type of antibody formation, but whether this is really worthwhile is also controversial.

Despite the fact that anti-TNFs are sometimes used to treat chronic skin diseases, the first appearance of psoriasis and other skin conditions has been reported to be a newly recognized side effect.

Anti-TNFs appear to increase the risk of lymphoma (lymph gland cancer). At the time of writing, although it is believed that this is a true risk, it is not completely certain since the majority of patients who have developed lymphoma were also being treated with immunosuppressives. See the Risk of Serious Events table on page 92, for the risk estimate.

Anti-integrins
NATALIZUMAB

Substances called cellular adhesion molecules (CAMs) regulate the entry of white blood cells into normal and inflamed segments of the intestine. CAMs cause certain white cells to adhere to the inner surfaces of blood vessels; once they are stuck there, they are able to move through the vessel wall and into the tissues of the gut wall, causing the inflammatory process. Some CAMs, such as alpha4 integrin, are

Risk of Serious Events

Serious Event	Annual Estimated Probability
Non-Hodgkin's lymphoma (baseline, all ages)	0.02% (2/10,000 patient-years)
Non-Hodgkin's lymphoma (on immunosuppressives)	0.04% (4/10,000 patient-years)
Non-Hodgkin's lymphoma (on anti-TNF)	0.06% (6/10,000 patient-years)[†]
Hepatosplenic T-cell lymphoma*	Unknown, but very rare so far
Death due to infection	0.4% (4/1,000 patient-years)
Active tuberculosis	0.05% (5/10,000 patient-years)

* A rare form of lymphoma, observed mainly in young men (under age 30) who are on both azathioprine or 6-mercaptopurine and anti-TNF therapy.
† Most people on anti-TNF therapy are also on immunosuppressives, and most of the excess lymphoma cases have been people with rheumatoid arthritis, and not IBD.

located on the surface of white blood cells, while others are on the surface of the blood vessels. In IBD, most of these CAMs are overactive. Natalizumab is an anti-alpha4 integrin antibody.

How Does It Work?
Natalizumab acts by preventing lymphocytes (a type of white blood cell) from sticking to the inner lining cells of the blood vessels. If they don't stick, they won't enter the surrounding tissues.

When Is It Used?
Like infliximab, natalizumab is given intravenously. Since its introduction in clinical trials, it has been on the market, off, and then back on (in some countries). Its main use has been in the disease multiple sclerosis (MS), but it has also been beneficial to people with IBD. Although it has provided dramatic remissions for some people with Crohn's disease who had failed anti-TNF drugs, it was found to cause a rare but lethal brain disease, known as progressive multifocal leuko-

encephalopathy (PML), which is due to a virus known as the JC virus. At the time of writing, this drug is back on the market; in some countries, the only approved indication is multiple sclerosis (MS), while in other countries, the drug can be given for both Crohn's and MS.

What Are the Side Effects?
Side effects include:

- headache;
- infusion reactions (fever, rash, flushing, nausea);
- mood change, including depression; and
- PML (see page 92) — similar to MS, but usually fatal.

Other Biologicals

Another anti-alpha4 integrin known as LDP-02 has been designed and tested in both ulcerative colitis and Crohn's disease, but progress has been slow. Vedolizumab is another biological currently being tested in clinical trials. Yet another biological, ustekinumab, has proven to be useful for psoriasis, but is less impressive in IBD so far.

Other Therapies

Growth Factors

GRANULOCYTE-MACROPHAGE COLONY-STIMULATING FACTOR
(GM-CSF) AND GRANULOCYTE COLONY-STIMULATING FACTOR
(G-CSF)

Growth factors are naturally occurring substances that are capable of stimulating cellular growth, proliferation and cellular differentiation. Our bodies contain many of these factors, helping to regulate the activities of the cells that make up our bodies. Anti-inflammatory effects were discovered in 1990s, and a few small studies in Crohn's were done in the 2000s. In addition to GM-CSF and G-CSF, other growth factors that appear promising for the treatment of IBD are keratinocyte-like growth factor-2 (KGF-2), epidermal growth factor (EGF) enemas used in combination with oral 5-ASA, and somatropin (human growth hormone).

Stem Cells

Human mesenchymal stem cells (hMSCs) are rare cells present in adult bone marrow with the capacity to differentiate into a variety of tissue types. We know that these cells are involved in the regulation of both immune and inflammatory responses. Bone marrow is readily available, and the technology to isolate and grow these cells has been developed. Furthermore, these cells have little or no effect on our immune system. All of this means that these cells can be the basis for the development of a new class of drugs and treatment. It appears that these cells can be transplanted without matching between donors and recipients. These features, along with our ability to produce and store these cells long term, have created considerable excitement for the future management of IBD. At present, however, this type of treatment is experimental and should be administered only in clinical trials. Such trials are underway.

Antibiotics

Over the years, various antibiotics have been used in the treatment of both ulcerative colitis and Crohn's disease. Antibiotics are not a primary therapy for ulcerative colitis but may be given along with other forms of therapy. However, they *may* be used as a primary therapy in Crohn's disease, with no other medication or treatment given.

ANTIBIOTICS IN ULCERATIVE COLITIS

Antibiotics alone are not a treatment for ulcerative colitis. The antibiotics used are generally classified as broad spectrum. This means they are effective against a large number of different bacteria. Commonly used antibiotics in this group are ampicillin, ceftriaxone, ciprofloxacin and metronidazole. Numerous other broad-spectrum antibiotics

---

Metronidazole and Alcohol

It was previously thought that anyone on metronidazole should avoid alcohol totally, but further experience has shown that not everyone reacts to this combination.

If you wish to drink, experiment first with very small amounts. If you want to drink beer, try just a mouthful, then two mouthfuls on another occasion, and so on. If you get to half a cup without a problem, it is very unlikely you will experience a reaction. Try even smaller amounts of stronger drinks: a small swallow of wine or a mere sip of liquor. Many patients prefer simply to avoid alcohol rather than risk being very ill from a reaction; however, people on long-term metronidazole who hope to resume responsible drinking can minimize the risk by this gradual approach.

are less commonly used, mainly because they are more expensive, without added benefits.

Some gastroenterologists prescribe antibiotics as part of the treatment of severe attacks. When the colon is badly inflamed, the bacteria normally present can easily penetrate the intestinal wall and move into the surrounding tissues and even the bloodstream. This can produce serious complications. Two of the most serious are septicemia (infected blood) and one or more abscesses (boils) in the liver. Doctors believe that giving antibiotic therapy while the attack of colitis is being treated in the usual way greatly reduces the risk of these complications.

ANTIBIOTICS IN CROHN'S DISEASE
It has been long known that antibiotics alone can be used to treat some patients with Crohn's disease. Various antibiotics have been used, including ampicillin, tetracycline, erythromycin, cephalexin and clarithromycin. The two most popular are metronidazole and ciprofloxacin.

Metronidazole

Metronidazole is particularly effective against a group of intestinal bacteria known as anaerobes — bacteria that do best in tissues where there is little or no oxygen. Metronidazole is used alone, or in combination with ciprofloxacin.

In Crohn's disease, the full thickness of the intestinal wall is inflamed. Little breaks can develop in the inner lining of the intestine, and these breaks can lead to little openings, called sinus tracts, that penetrate through the wall of the bowel into the surrounding tissues. These sinus tracts frequently result in abscesses, and sometimes fistulas as well (see Chapter 9). Metronidazole is particularly useful in the treatment of abscesses (boils) and fistulas at or near the anus. It is available as capsules, tablets, a cream or in an injectable form.

Metronidazole has been shown to benefit some people with Crohn's colitis. Someone who has not responded to sulfasalazine may respond to metronidazole; however, someone who has not responded to metronidazole is unlikely to respond to sulfasalazine. Metronidazole is sometimes used to treat small bowel Crohn's disease, although the benefit has not been proven. It does not prevent acute attacks; however, studies have shown that it can delay, and possibly decrease, recurrence of the disease after surgery.

SIDE EFFECTS OF METRONIDAZOLE

By far the most common side effects of metronidazole are gastrointestinal. Nausea, decreased appetite, vomiting, constipation, diarrhea and indigestion have all been reported, though only the first two are relatively common. Some patients complain of a constant metallic taste in the mouth. Others find that everything they eat tastes bad. The tongue may feel or even appear "furry," with a brownish coating. Continuous therapy for weeks to months can damage the nerves in the feet and legs. This shows up as persistent numbness or tingling in the feet, or difficulty with balance (clumsiness or unsteadiness), especially when walking. These effects are generally reversible, though the return to normal may take several months after the drug has been stopped.

Headaches can occur but are more likely in association with alcohol. Although most interactions with alcohol are related to drinking alcoholic beverages, sometimes someone gets headaches simply by absorbing alcohol through the skin from perfumes or colognes.

Some people who drink alcohol while on metronidazole become quite ill. Symptoms include extreme flushing of the face, shortness of breath, severe headache, rapid and pounding heartbeat, nausea and vomiting and, occasionally, collapse. Recovery is complete following a period of drowsiness or sleep. (See Metronidazole and Alcohol on page 94.)

Ciprofloxacin

Although few controlled studies have been done, there have been several enthusiastic reports about this antibiotic, alone or in combination with metronidazole, in people with perianal Crohn's disease. It is also used to treat some cases of Crohn's ileitis or colitis, or both.

SIDE EFFECTS OF CIPROFLOXACIN

This drug is very well tolerated. The most common side effects are nausea and diarrhea, which occur in only about one in a hundred patients. Ciprofloxacin slows down the inactivation of caffeine, prolonging and possibly increasing its stimulant effect. This does not mean that caffeine should be avoided, just that people who are sensitive to its stimulating effects should be aware of this possible increase. Some individuals have reported difficulty sleeping and vivid dreams. Drugs in this class can also cause inflammation of tendons (tendonitis), and there are reports of ruptured (torn) tendons, particularly the Achilles tendon.

Probiotics and Prebiotics

We are born germ-free, but our gastrointestinal system rapidly becomes colonized by bacteria and other germs from our food and environment. Some of these, known as probiotic or "friendly" bacteria, appear to play a role in keeping us healthy. When we eat foods with friendly bacteria (such as yogurt containing active culture), they may help replace "unfriendly" bacteria that may be making us ill.

Antibiotics can upset the normal bacterial population of our gastrointestinal system. Once these drugs are stopped, our bodies may not be able to restore the normal bacteria, especially if we are malnourished. Probiotics *seem* to help, in some cases.

Many nonfood probiotic products are on the market; unfortunately, their quality control tends to be poor and their safety cannot be guaranteed. There are a few quality-controlled products available, but at present they are fairly expensive.

There are also foods and nutrients known as prebiotics, which the friendly bacteria need to maintain themselves. Honey, onions, inulin and some grains are examples of foods containing prebiotics.

Although there have been several studies using probiotics for IBD, and many claims of benefit, so far the only really convincing study is one that showed VSL-3 to be effective in controlling pouchitis (see Chapter 7). A bacterial strain known as E. coli Nissle 1917 has produced some interesting results in maintenance of remission in ulcerative colitis, but further study is needed, and more studies are underway. Karen Madsen, a Canadian researcher, has put forth the concept that it is highly probable that we need to use different probiotics for different medical conditions, just as we need different antibiotics for different infections.

Fish Oil

Naturally occurring chemicals known as omega-3 fatty acids have been shown to have anti-inflammatory properties. One source of these chemicals is fish oil.

There is one controlled study in people with Crohn's disease that showed that more people on fish oil stayed in remission compared with those on a placebo, and there is one, more recent, controlled study showing no benefit. A few studies have been done in ulcerative colitis, some showing a modest short-term benefit, while others show no benefit. Fish oil may also help some people with arthritis, so if you have both IBD and arthritis you may receive a double benefit. Note that if you take what is considered a therapeutic amount of fish oil, you may end up smelling like fish! While this side effect is clearly not serious, it is certainly undesirable. Other side effects, which are uncommon, include nausea and diarrhea. If you are going to try this, look for a product that contains 180 milligrams of eicosapentanoic acid (EPA) and 120 milligrams of docosahexanoic acid (DHA).

Lidocaine Enemas

We've known for many years that chronic bowel inflammation causes enlargement of nerve cells within the bowel wall. Researchers discovered that these nerve cells release chemicals that promote inflammation by attracting white blood cells. A Scandinavian doctor came up with the idea of putting local anesthetic into the rectums of people with ulcerative colitis. In theory, "freezing" the nerves would prevent these chemicals from being released and would stop the inflammation. No one has had the success rates this doctor claimed, but some people do respond to lidocaine enemas.

There is no lidocaine enema on the market. Tubes of this jelly come with a little screw-on plastic tip, which can be used to deliver the medication into the rectum, but some people will find the tip too short and will need a catheter-tip syringe. Don't use this treatment unless it's prescribed by your doctor. The usual dose is 30 milliliters daily; most drug plans don't pay for it.

When used in other ways, lidocaine can cause epileptic seizures if absorbed into the bloodstream in large quantities. However, this side effect has not been reported with enema therapy. Other than that, there do not seem to be any side effects of using lidocaine in this way.

Heparin

In 1991, Dr. P. Gaffney, an Irish physician, reported an ulcerative colitis patient who needed the anticoagulant (blood thinner) heparin for a blood clot in his leg. His colitis, which was not responding very well to treatment, improved dramatically when the heparin was started. Although several studies have verified that this treatment seems to work in some patients, especially if the patient is on sulfasalazine, heparin is really not part of standard therapy at present. However, it is useful to know that we can use this drug in colitis patients who require anticoagulation. Heparin and its newer forms (low molecular weight heparin) have anti-inflammatory properties. Studies are continuing with newer heparin derivatives.

Nicotine

Nicotine protects some people against ulcerative colitis.

Statistics from many IBD centers have shown that there are three times as many nonsmokers as smokers with ulcerative colitis. Studies have also shown that it is not the act of stopping smoking that increases the risk; rather, it is simply the fact of becoming a nonsmoker. This means that a person who quits smoking has the same risk of developing colitis as a person who has never smoked. Nicotine is the active ingredient.

How nicotine protects against ulcerative colitis is unknown. The therapeutic effect can be achieved by smoking but, considering the health hazards of smoking, this is obviously not a reasonable strategy. Nicotine-containing gum has been used, but it is not popular because it is very sticky and hard to chew. It is better tolerated if sucked, but this is difficult to do for prolonged periods. The nicotine patch has made this therapy more practical.

However, nicotine patches are expensive, and many drug plans will not pay for this form of treatment. People who have never smoked may be less likely to tolerate nicotine than those who have. Only brief (6-week) studies have been done. We don't know if long-term use of nicotine in this way is safe or effective. The most common side effects include nausea, light-headedness, headache, sleep disturbance or vivid dreams, dizziness, skin irritation due to the patch, sweating, and trembling hands.

If you have Crohn's disease, take note. Smoking may be protective for some people with ulcerative colitis, but it is bad for some people with Crohn's. If you do smoke, note that stopping smoking is beneficial to some people with Crohn's.

Other Drugs for IBD

It is beyond the scope of this book to cover all the treatments for IBD described in the literature. Some of the ones still under study are LDP-02, anti-TB drug combinations, alicaforsen enemas, teduglutide, autologous protein-containing colon extract, extracorporeal photochemotherapy (also known as photopheresis), CCX 282, naltrexone and some herbal products.

Drugs That Reduce Symptoms without Affecting Inflammation

Certain drugs do not reduce inflammation but are used to reduce or eliminate symptoms.

ANTIDIARRHEALS

During IBD flare-ups, most gastroenterologists prefer that you avoid these drugs because complications may be more likely to occur. But between flare-ups, many patients, especially those with Crohn's disease, are troubled by urgency, cramps and diarrhea. Until and unless these symptoms can be controlled by specific treatments that eliminate inflammation, these symptoms may be controlled with antidiarrheal drugs, which are generally quite safe. Furthermore, these drugs can make a huge quality-of-life difference for people with bile-salt diarrhea (see Chapter 7), short bowel syndrome or a high-output stoma.

How do antidiarrheal drugs work? Antidiarrheal drugs work by altering the muscle activity of the small and large intestines, causing waste material to pass through more slowly, and allowing more water to be absorbed, resulting in more solid bowel movements. Contraction strength of the bowel wall muscle is also reduced, and this prevents, or reduces, crampy abdominal pain.

What are the side effects? When taken between IBD flare-ups, the main side effect of antidiarrheal drugs is constipation, which may in turn increase abdominal pain and cause a sensation of bloating. Do not take these drugs if you think you are having a flare-up or an obstruction unless advised to do so by your doctor.

The narcotic antidiarrheal medications (codeine and diphenoxylate) may also cause nausea, vomiting, drowsiness, dizziness and itchy rashes. However, these are all very uncommon. All narcotics carry the risk of addiction, but the risk is extremely low when these drugs are used in the treatment of bowel disorders.

Loperamide is the safest of all the antidiarrheal drugs and is often the first choice when an antidiarrheal drug is needed. It is chemically similar to the narcotics but is not classified as one and is therefore available over the counter, without a prescription. One drawback is that most private drug plans will not pay for it. In Canada, some provincial plans will pay for it, provided your doctor indicates that it is for treatment of IBD, or for someone with an ostomy. However, if cost is an issue, a drug that is covered by your plan may be prescribed instead.

Not only is loperamide the safest antidiarrheal drug, but it is also long-acting, so that it usually needs to be taken only one to three times a day. In comparison, diphenoxylate and codeine usually need to be taken three to five times a day. The fewer times a medication has to be taken, the more likely it is to be taken at the right times. Loperamide, diphenoxylate and codeine are all available as tablets, and loperamide and codeine are also available as syrups.

BULK FORMERS
Bulk formers are drugs that soak up water in the stool, reducing looseness and sometimes frequency of stools as well. They may be thought of as commercial forms of fiber.

When are they used? Relatively mild diarrhea in both ulcerative colitis and Crohn's disease can sometimes be controlled with bulk formers. However, bear in mind that while the stools may be more solid, they may also be more frequent, rather than less frequent.

What are the side effects? Side effects with bulk formers are very uncommon. Some individuals feel bloated and gassy. Many products give off a fine dust when they are handled; inhaling this dust repeatedly can cause you to become allergic, and serious reactions may result. But this is extremely rare. You can avoid this by handling the products at arm's length.

Bulk formers are sold in many flavors, as powders or granules. Most are some form of psyllium, a natural fiber source. Wheat bran can be equally effective.

BILE-SALT BINDERS
These drugs bind (form a chemical complex) with bile salts, a normal product of the liver. Bile salts flow, dissolved in the bile, from the liver via the bile duct to the intestine, where they aid in digesting fat.

Normally, 90 to 99 percent of the bile salts are reabsorbed by the ileum and recycled. The 1 to 10 percent that reaches the colon is lost in the stool without causing any problems. However, if some of the ileum is diseased or has been removed, more of the bile salts reach the colon. The excess irritates the lining of the colon. This causes an outpouring of water into the colon, which is the opposite of what is supposed to happen (normally water is absorbed). The result is diarrhea. By forming a chemical complex with the bile salts, bile-salt binders can prevent this form of diarrhea.

When are they used? Diarrhea in someone with ileal disease or previous ileal resection (see Chapter 7) can be treated with these drugs. However, diarrhea that is equally well controlled by one of the other antidiarrheals is perfectly acceptable medically, and may well be more acceptable to the person. These drugs are generally not used in ulcerative colitis.

What are the side effects? People on bile-salt binders may have difficulty digesting and absorbing fat. This occurs mainly in those who have extensive ileal disease or who have had a surgical resection (removal) of more than 3 feet (about 1 meter) of ileum. The vitamins A, D, E and K are all fats and therefore may not be absorbed normally. This can generally be treated with vitamin supplements. These vitamins can be toxic; do not take them in large amounts without consulting your doctor.

Other side effects of bile-salt binders include nausea, vomiting, constipation, abdominal pain and bloating. Occasionally, folate (a B vitamin) deficiency develops due to decreased absorption. Absorption of other medications taken at the same time may be reduced or delayed. Cholestyramine is the only antidiarrheal bile-salt binder currently available. It comes as a powder that doesn't really dissolve in anything, and it has a metallic taste. Because cholestyramine powder is inconvenient and unpalatable, many physicians (and patients) prefer to use loperamide, diphenoxylate or codeine for bile-salt diarrhea, even though cholestyramine is theoretically more specific.

Other Conditions and Treatments
Hemorrhoids and Anal Fissures

What Can I Take for Constipation During a Colitis Flare-up?

For people with mild colitis involving the last 2 feet (about 0.5 meter) or less of the colon. It is essential that you check with your doctor before following any of these suggestions.

If you have been constipated for 4 days or less, taking a laxative, such as milk of magnesia or PEG 3350, or giving yourself a small enema of plain tap water may be all that is necessary. An alternative is to use a glycerin suppository or, for something with a little more punch, a bisacodyl suppository.

If a laxative, suppository or enema does not "uncork" the system, or if you've been constipated for more than 4 days, you generally must take something by mouth to thoroughly soften and flush out the accumulated stool. The first and safest choice is to drink 1 or 2 liters of a colonic lavage solution. These solutions are mildly salty and contain polyethylene glycol, or PEG. The PEG prevents the salt and water from being absorbed into the blood, and the result is that the colon is flushed out. Some colonic lavage solutions are flavored. I advise my patients to drink about 0.5 liter (two 8-ounce cups) an hour, or to take it even more slowly if nausea is a problem. (These directions are different from those on the container; see Chapter 4.) The second choice (which has risks for some people) is to mix and drink a packet of a sodium picosulfate product. If you choose sodium picosulfate, you must drink as much clear fluid — at least 1 quart (1 liter) of juices or broths — as possible for the next 5 hours; then you can resume eating. If you don't drink enough fluid, you will become dehydrated. Bowel movements will usually begin in about 2 hours, and most people will be cleaned out within about 5 hours. Whatever the product used, some people will not tolerate it. A packet of picosulfate solution is roughly equivalent to 2 liters of PEG–salt water solution. Whichever method you use, it is not necessary to achieve the total cleanout needed before a colonoscopy or barium enema. If the attack of colitis has been controlled, the constipation will probably not come back.

Some people should not or cannot drink either of these but do need something for the constipation that can occur during an attack of colitis. You should avoid harsh laxatives. This includes most over-the-counter brand-name laxatives. My suggestion in this situation is to take mineral oil. (A raspberry-flavored brand is available in some countries.) Take 2 tablespoons (30 milliliters) every 2 to 4 hours during your normal waking hours. Eat normally. Typically after about 2 days, you will start to pass some oil from the rectum. (You may want to put a pad or some tissue in your underwear to soak up the oil.) Continue the same dose of oil until you have had 2 or 3 large, greasy bowel movements, or 10 or more smaller ones. Then reduce the oil to 1 tablespoon (15 milliliters) a day, in the evening, until it is clear that the attack of colitis is coming under control. At this point, you can stop the oil. The constipation should not come back. ☛

Mineral oil is undesirable as a laxative on a regular basis. It is messy and inconvenient. Some physicians believe it can interfere with absorption of the fat-soluble vitamins (A, D, E and K), but this is unproven.

Everyone has little veins in the anal canal, called the hemorrhoidal veins. The term "hemorrhoids" refers to enlargement of one or more of these veins. Hemorrhoids usually develop as a result of pushing hard to have bowel movements, or sometimes just because of frequent bowel movements. Hemorrhoids that are not bleeding and not causing any other problems don't require any treatment. When hemorrhoids do need to be treated, the treatment is much the same as it is for anal fissures (see Chapter 9). If bowel movements are hard, something needs to be done to make them softer. As you can imagine, the words "hard" and "soft" mean different things to different people. A misunderstanding between a doctor and a patient can lead to making the stools excessively soft. This can be a problem because excessive softening is usually associated with increased frequency, and that is often not desirable. When your IBD is well controlled, you should aim for one or two large, formed, easy-to-pass bowel movements every day, if possible, without forcing or straining. Many people can achieve this simply by increasing the amount of fiber in their diet.

In addition to regular bowel movements, it is useful to apply local medication to reduce inflammation in the area of the hemorrhoids or fissures, or both. The things that work best are ointments and suppositories that contain a very small amount of a steroid, usually hydrocortisone. Both bowel regularity and local steroid medication shrink the tissues around hemorrhoids and reduce the overall swelling.

Reducing inflammation is a particularly important part of treating fissures. Inflammation in the region of the anus usually causes some spasm (excessive and persistent muscular activity) of the anal sphincter. This promotes constipation because passing stool is resisted. Constipation temporarily makes things better because the fissure can start to heal or hemorrhoids can start to shrink when nothing is passing through the anal canal and no attempt is being made to pass anything. However, whenever the sufferer then has a bowel movement, the whole problem is aggravated because forcing and straining *will* be necessary and the stool that comes out will be excessively hard or large in diameter, or both.

Applying a steroid-containing ointment locally and regulating the stool are frequently adequate to treat hemorrhoids but sometimes not enough to treat fissures. The main goal of treating anal fissures is to relax the anal sphincter. One of the simplest and most effective things you can do to relax the anal sphincter is to use a sitz bath at least once a day. A sitz bath is a plastic bowl that looks much like a bedpan. It fits into your toilet and has a flange around it that rests on the edge of the bowl. The sitz bath has little overflow holes so that water in the pan does not spill onto the floor when you sit in it. All you need to do is fill it with plain warm water; you don't have to add salt or baking soda. Be careful to avoid using water that is too hot, as burning the skin will simply injure and inflame it further. Five to 10 minutes per sitz bath is enough. Sitz baths are best right after a bowel movement, but many people find that the most convenient time is at bedtime. If you happen to have a bidet in your bathroom, you can use it instead.

Fissures resistant to the above treatments are sometimes treated with nitroglycerine ointment (there is no commercial product; it is usually manufactured in hospital pharmacies), diltiazem or nifedipine ointment or botulinum toxin injection. Space does not permit detailed discussion of these therapies; check with your physician. You should not use steroid-containing ointments or suppositories indefinitely because one of the long-term side effects is a thinning of the skin, so it will actually become less resistant to irritation. Once the acute problem has subsided, continue with bowel regulation and sitz baths as needed.

Many people with IBD are troubled by hemorrhoids or fissures as a result of chronic diarrhea rather than constipation. High-fiber diets are *not* usually helpful in reducing diarrhea. Your doctor is the person to consult for the best treatment of diarrhea, be it through some change in your diet or through medication.

Itching in or around the Anus
Another complaint frequently associated with hemorrhoids is an itch in the region of the anus. This usually occurs for one of two reasons. The skin of the anal canal first becomes irritated because of frequent wiping. Once the skin is irritated, it becomes even more sensitive than usual. Stool is irritating to skin. Even when people are quite careful

about wiping themselves, bits of stool are frequently left between the multiple folds of skin present in the anal canal. If you have hemorrhoids, there are even more folds where bits of stool can get trapped. The stool further inflames the already irritated skin. This results in an itch. This is not serious but can be a major nuisance, especially at night, when your brain is not distracted.

The treatment for an anal itch is much the same as the treatment for hemorrhoids and fissures. Controlling diarrhea is important so you won't have to wipe frequently. Cleaning the skin through the use of sitz baths is helpful because no rubbing is necessary. When you sit in the sitz bath, the anal sphincter relaxes, releasing bits of stool trapped between the folds of the anal lining. It is often helpful to apply some kind of ointment to the irritated area after the sitz bath. Initially this can be a steroid-containing ointment. Eventually what will be needed is simply something to act as a barrier to protect the skin against further irritation by stool. Zinc oxide, various baby ointments and even petroleum jelly are all acceptable. If itching is an ongoing or frequently recurring problem, changing your toilet habits may help. After wiping off most of the residual stool following a bowel movement, fold some toilet paper, wet it, then press it onto the area around the anus. Doing this two or three times will enable you to complete cleaning the area without any rubbing. If you have diarrhea and must do this frequently, the skin will get quite dry. In this situation, apply a barrier ointment of some kind (I usually recommend petroleum jelly) every night. If an anal itch is intense or resistant to treatment, there may be another cause. Consult your doctor.

OSTEOPOROSIS

Osteoporosis is a disease of the skeleton that is characterized by decreased bone strength. This means that your bones break more easily. It is especially common in the spine. Millions of people have this condition. Increasing age, race and gender all contribute to the development of osteoporosis, but nutritional and lifestyle risk factors can also contribute.

People with IBD are more susceptible to osteoporosis than the general population. Risk factors in IBD patients include chronic or frequent steroid therapy, a low-lactose diet, malnutrition, lack of exercise because of illness, and lack of vitamin D (due to geographic location or decreased absorption, or both). The best strategy is prevention, but this is not always possible. Many people already have this condition when they are first diagnosed with IBD.

The ideal treatment of osteoporosis involves drugs, calcium and vitamin D supplementation, and an exercise program. Being able to reduce, stop or avoid steroids is helpful. But the most important factor is often control of your IBD; chronic inflammatory diseases appear to interfere with the body's mechanisms for maintaining bone health. While active IBD is present, we often stabilize osteoporosis; when the disease is removed surgically, or when we achieve healing of the disease, the bones often improve with treatment, sometimes right back to normal.

Commonly used drugs for osteoporosis include alendronate, risedronate, calcitonin nasal spray and teriparatide injections (this drug is used mainly for severe osteoporosis). Sometimes the first two are combined with calcium or vitamin D.

Common side effects of these drugs are as follows:

- Alendronate and risedronate (also known as bisphosphonates): most commonly, ulceration of the esophagus, causing heartburn or chest pain; these medications should always be taken with at least 6 ounces of water and *never* when lying down.
- Calcitonin: back pain, joint pain, headaches and nasal irritation, with runny nose, or dryness, crusting and, sometimes, bleeding.
- Teriparatide: constipation, diarrhea, headache, indigestion, cough, joint pain, leg or back cramps and injection site reactions, including one or more of the following: minor bruising, itching, pain, redness and swelling.

For information on how to achieve healthy bones, see Chapter 12.

Analgesics (Painkillers)

Occasionally, you may feel you need a painkiller for symptoms not controlled by your regular medications, or for some unrelated problem — a headache, for example.

ASA, the most widely available nonprescription painkiller, is somewhat undesirable in IBD. Its chemical properties make ulcerative colitis patients bleed more when the colon is inflamed. Stomach and duodenal ulcers are more common in Crohn's disease patients than in the general population, and ASA increases the risk of getting an ulcer.

The preferred nonprescription analgesic is acetaminophen; it is available under many names, but generic or no-name forms are just as good. Acetaminophen also has risks, but for the IBD patient it does not have as many as ASA. An overdose of acetaminophen can fatally injure the liver. Large doses taken for many years may cause kidney damage.

Nonsteroidal Anti-inflammatory Drugs (NSAIDs)

Some 10 to 20 percent of people with IBD experience pain in one or more joints. In some cases, simple acetaminophen is enough to relieve the pain. However, many people require drugs specifically for arthritis. These all fall into a family known as nonsteroidal anti-inflammatory drugs (NSAIDs), commonly referred to as anti-inflammatories. These are currently divided into three groups: nonselective, partially selective and selective (also known as coxibs).

Drugs in the first group include ibuprofen, indomethacin, naproxen, sulindac, piroxicam, ketoprofen, ketorolac and diclofenac, among others. Drugs in the partially selective group include meloxicam, etodolac and nabumetone. There used to be a long list of drugs in the selective group, including celecoxib, rofecoxib, valdecoxib, etoricoxib and others. However, all except celecoxib have been taken off the market because of cardiac risks.

Any of these drugs can occasionally cause inflammation of the colon (so-called NSAID colitis). This reaction is no more likely to occur in people with IBD than in those without it. It usually gets better quickly when the drug is stopped. However, there is also a small chance that a reaction to the drug will trigger an IBD flare-up. While this risk is real, the extent of this risk has been greatly overestimated in the past. This is not an allergic reaction, and it does not mean that NSAIDs must be avoided. In fact, it is not even clearly established that the same drug will cause the same reaction if it is taken again on another occasion. It appears that this reaction is less likely with selective NSAIDs.

SIDE EFFECTS OF NSAIDS

As well as the side effects discussed above, up to 25 percent of people taking NSAIDs experience burning discomfort in the upper abdomen or behind the breastbone (heartburn), or some other form of indigestion. People with a history of acid-related problems and people over 60 are much more prone to this, and a protective drug should be prescribed. The risk of ulcers in the stomach or duodenum from taking these medications can be reduced by using misoprostol at the same time, but a common side effect of *that* drug, when taken in the proper dose, is diarrhea. Better protection with fewer side effects is achieved with proton pump inhibitors such as omeprazole, panto-prazole, lansoprazole, rabeprazole, esomeprazole or dexlansoprazole. The risk of ulcers is much less with selective NSAIDs, and protection may not be needed. Check with your doctor. Other relatively common side effects are nausea and allergic reactions.

Some NSAIDs come in slow-release forms or are long-acting and can be taken once or twice a day. Others need to be taken three or four times a day. The slow-release forms can cause ulceration and even perforation of the small intestine and colon. Because at least one of those areas is already abnormal in someone with IBD, there may be a greater risk of this happening, especially in people with strictures of the small bowel.

Although some people must take these drugs continuously for months or even years, using them intermittently is preferable, if possible. Except for ankylosing spondylitis (see Chapter 9), most arthritis associated with IBD does not damage or destroy joints, so getting rid of the inflammation is not essential. See if you can control minor aches and pains with acetaminophen, which is considerably safer.

Antibiotics

As discussed earlier, some antibiotics may be used to treat people with Crohn's disease. But you might also need antibiotics for other conditions. It is comforting to know that antibiotics are no more likely to cause adverse effects in people with IBD than in other individuals. They should be prescribed and taken when needed. But remember that antibiotics occasionally cause a form of colitis due to an over-growth of the bacterium Clostridium difficile ("C. diff" for short). It's usually fairly easy to distinguish between colitis due to IBD and antibiotic-associated colitis, though. If you are having an attack of colitis, *always* tell your gastroenterologist if you are on antibiotics or have been within the past few months.

Acid-reducing Drugs

Heartburn, a burning sensation felt behind the breastbone or in the upper abdomen just below the breastbone, is usually due to a condition called reflux esophagitis, in which stomach acid backs up into the esophagus. Millions of people around the world have it, including many people with IBD. The most effective therapy is to reduce the amount of acid produced by the stomach. All the drugs in the acid-reducing category have few side effects and can be taken with any of the standard therapies for IBD.

The best-known acid-reducing drugs are in one of two families. The first group is known as histamine-2-receptor antagonists (or H-2 blockers). They include cimetidine, ranitidine, famotidine and nizatidine. The second group is called proton pump inhibitors, or PPIs. These include omeprazole, pantoprazole, lansoprazole, rabeprazole, esomeprazole and dexlansoprazole. The PPIs are the most potent acid-suppressing medications we have. However, they are also the most expensive and are not always necessary. Stomach acid has the important protective function of killing the germs we take in with food. Therefore, suppressing the production of acid just enough to relieve your symptoms may be preferable. However, if your doctor feels you need a PPI, do not switch to a less potent medication without discussing it.

Erythropoietin

Chronic diseases can suppress bone marrow function so that even if all the building blocks (one of them being iron; see below) are available, red blood cell production may be reduced. (This condition is called anemia.) Erythropoietin is a natural substance that stimulates red blood cell production. In a small number of patients with IBD, erythropoietin may be helpful in treating anemia when providing the building blocks such as iron, folic acid or vitamin B12 is not enough. You may feel more energetic, but there is no effect on the disease itself.

Iron

Iron-deficiency anemia is a common problem in IBD (see Chapter 9). If it develops, most patients will require supplemental iron.

Iron tablets come in many forms. Commonly used products include ferrous sulfate, ferrous fumarate and ferrous gluconate. Common side effects of taking iron supplements are nausea and a change in bowel

Advantages and Disadvantages of Iron Injections

Intramuscular:
- given at the doctor's office;
- should be given into large muscle mass;
- multiple injections are necessary;
- immediate side effects include pain at the injection site and allergic reactions, occasionally severe;
- risk of side effects increased if iron pills are also being taken.

Intravenous:
- a large muscle mass is not necessary (some IBD patients are underweight);
- not painful;
- multiple doses usually necessary;
- immediate side effects are mainly due to rapid infusion; include pain, swelling and redness at injection site;
- usually given in hospital or clinic setting.

The most important thing about receiving iron injections, either intramuscularly or intravenously, is to be sure that this form of supplementation is truly necessary.

habit. Some people get diarrhea; others get constipated. Sometimes these side effects cause enough trouble that the dose has to be reduced or the medication even stopped. All patients on supplemental iron notice that their stools are darker and may even appear black. This is because much of the iron in each pill is not absorbed.

If you have unacceptable side effects with even one iron tablet a day, try a combination of a small amount of an iron-containing syrup and a high-iron diet (see Appendix 5). If you cannot get enough iron by mouth, you'll have to get it by injection, either intramuscularly (into muscle) or intravenously (into a vein). Although it may be more convenient for you to go to your doctor's office and get an intramuscular injection of iron, such injections are often painful and have to be given frequently. There is an excellent intravenous iron product named ferrous saccharate. You have to attend a hospital outpatient clinic or some other clinic setting to receive this. Most people require two or three intravenous infusions to get the total amount of iron that they need. Side effects are extremely uncommon.

Absorption of iron from medication or food is very limited. Your doctor can monitor the need with blood tests. Do not take iron pills or high-iron foods indefinitely without your doctor's agreement.

Calcium

If your calcium intake is below the recommended daily amount (see Appendix 3), you can improve your intake either by changing your diet or by taking calcium tablets, or both. If you are going to take calcium tablets, *tell your doctor.* Calcium is absorbed more effectively in the presence of vitamin D. You can buy a calcium–vitamin D tablet. Remember that both vitamin D and calcium can be bad for you, as well as good for you. Too much of either one can make you seriously ill. Just because a little vitamin D is needed to help absorb calcium doesn't mean that a lot is better for you. However, if you live in a part of the world where the sun is low in the sky and the days are short for several months a year, it is likely that you need extra vitamin D even if you don't need to take extra calcium. A simple blood test can measure your vitamin D level. Discuss this with your doctor.

Some people get constipated on calcium and this may mean the dose has to be reduced. Taking excessive calcium can lead to kidney stones, and even calcium deposits in various organs and tissues, sometimes with serious results.

Numerous calcium tablets are available on the market. Some are name brand; many sold in large chain pharmacies are house brand; and there are others. Some calcium products are derived from oyster shells or dolomite, which may be contaminated with arsenic or other undesirable substances. Name brand and large chain pharmacy house brand calcium tablets are preferable.

Some people take bone-meal tablets. These often contain powdered bone from animal bones, some of which contain a lot of lead. Such tablets are not an advisable source of calcium.

People on low-lactose diets may need a calcium supplement. For more information, see Chapter 5.

Zinc

Chronic diarrhea sometimes results in deficiencies of elements needed in trace amounts by the body. Some patients who have just gotten over an IBD flare-up have trouble gaining back weight they have lost. In some of these cases, taking a zinc supplement two or three times

Complementary and Alternative Therapies

The term "complementary" is usually used for treatments such as massage, tai chi, relaxation techniques and the like. Complementary therapies that help you feel more relaxed, stronger and more in control of your life are helpful and safe.

The label "alternative" is generally used to describe treatments based on naturopathy, homeopathy or related fields. While alternative medicine clearly helps some people feel better, be careful when such treatments involve prescription of herbs or other "natural" products. *Anything* that you take for health reasons is a drug.

It is important to realize that herbal drugs are simply drugs that come from plants. Digoxin, the heart medication, comes from the foxglove plant; taxol, a very valuable drug for ovarian cancer, comes from the Pacific yew tree; vincristine, a drug for leukemia, comes from the vinca plant; and ASA was originally an extract of willow bark. In other words, there is nothing exclusive about the use of medicines derived from plants.

But there are important differences between most herbal products and conventional drugs derived from plants. Conventional drugs are purified and studied carefully before being approved by regulatory agencies. Side-effect profiles are established. Because we know that new side effects, undetected during premarket testing, can still arise, there are ongoing surveillance and reporting mechanisms to protect the public as much as possible. This arrangement is not perfect, but our desire for absolute safety must be balanced by our need for better treatments for many diseases.

With most herbal products, you don't know if what's on the label is what's in the bottle, and you don't know if what's in the bottle is pure. For example, a few years ago kelp products were popular. Some of them turned out to contain significant amounts of arsenic, and there were several cases of arsenic poisoning. Among other risks, liver cancer can result from excessive intake of arsenic.

But the most important issue is that of safety. You should assume that anything that can benefit you may also have risks (side effects). Because (at the time of writing) there is little government regulation requiring makers of herbal products to test their products scientifically, we simply don't know the risks of taking most herbal products.

This does not mean that such products can't help some people; it's just that you can't assume they are safe because someone tells you they are. Over the years, many herbal products have been taken off the market after serious, sometimes fatal, side effects were discovered. The good news is that government agencies in several countries are starting to regulate "health-food" products and other herbal remedies, so that you and your medical team will be able to start to explore the therapeutic value of these products.

a day for a couple of weeks will facilitate weight gain. I usually prescribe elemental zinc tablets (50 milligrams each); the dose is one tablet three times a day for 2 weeks. If it doesn't help, taking it for longer is not usually worthwhile. Some people with zinc deficiency have a reduced sense of taste; once again, 2 weeks of treatment with zinc tablets can sometimes restore normal taste.

Vitamins

Many patients ask, "Do I need vitamin pills?" When the diet is restricted in some way for prolonged periods (such as several days of clear fluids in the hospital), some vitamin supplementation may be advisable. If you know you are eating poorly, take a one-a-day mineral preparation (tablet or liquid). Don't use products that contain other substances or amounts over the recommended daily allowance. I advise patients to buy house-brand products.

What about vitamin D? As mentioned above, if you live in a part of the world where the sun is low in the sky and the days are short for several months a year, you may need extra vitamin D. If possible, get your doctor to measure your 25-hydroxy vitamin D level. If you start taking a supplement, remember that for every 1,000 international units of vitamin D, your blood level goes up 25 units.

See Chapter 7 for a detailed discussion on vitamin B12.

People on an enteral diet and those on total parenteral nutrition (see Chapters 5 and 12) usually receive adequate amounts of both vitamins and minerals.

"Miracles" and Myths: The Placebo Effect

Characteristically, most chronic inflammatory diseases may get better or worse on their own. This can make any treatment look effective or ineffective. For this reason, carefully controlled studies are desirable. When patients are seriously ill, doctors cannot ethically give some of them a placebo (a substance known to have no therapeutic effect) if proven therapies are available. However, there are many situations in which temporarily withholding active treatment is acceptable, especially in the context of controlled clinical trials.

Such studies have taught us that, over a 4-month period, 25 to 40 percent of Crohn's patients with symptoms worthy of treatment gradually get better without specific active therapy. About 20 percent of these patients remain well for 1 year, and 10 percent stay well for 2 years. In addition, many patients whose disease is brought under control with active therapy remain well off treatment for 1 or 2 years or more. Findings are similar for people with ulcerative colitis. People receiving placebos may feel better for psychological reasons; if they think they are receiving a real treatment, they want it to work, and this positive attitude may be beneficial.

Whenever the cause of a chronic, incurable disease is unknown, you can expect all sorts of treatments and "cures" to be promoted. Some will be touted by people who really believe in what they are promoting. Other treatments are put forward by individuals or groups trying to make a buck. When people are both ill and poorly informed, they may become desperate, and this makes them susceptible to being taken in.

Unorthodox Therapies

Over the years, claims of dramatic success have been made for a wide variety of unorthodox therapies, sometimes on the basis of scanty reliable information.

In the 1970s, two researchers in New York maintained that a protein isolated from the pituitary gland of cows could control diarrhea in patients with Crohn's disease. In the 1980s, a company in the United States promoted a product made from the ground-up tracheas (windpipes) of cows. In the late 1980s, two researchers in Canada claimed that a naturally occurring compound known as N-acetyl glucosamine was beneficial to patients with inflammatory bowel disease. Some people have asserted that patients with IBD can be greatly helped by orthomolecular medicine, meaning treatment with multiple vitamins and minerals.

Until the true causes of IBD are known, unorthodox treatments will continue to be promoted. Because of the placebo effect, we should insist on carefully controlled, scientifically sound studies to evaluate any new proposed treatments, and view unsubstantiated claims with great suspicion. Anything that has biological activity is likely also to have biological risk. The idea that avoiding standard therapies means avoiding risk is faulty. When you need treatment and you avoid it, there is a significant risk that the disease or complication will get worse and may even endanger your life. By all means participate in your care. But do it in conjunction with your doctor.

7

Surgery for IBD

Many people think of surgery for inflammatory bowel disease as a last resort. Except for a few cases, it is not. Surgery is one of the important forms of treatment for IBD. Sometimes it's the best choice. Sometimes it's the only choice.

Using technical terms is unavoidable when discussing the various operations. Let's define some of the most common ones. You can also refer to the glossary at the back of the book.

In medical terminology, the suffix "ectomy" means removal. A colectomy is removal of the colon. Total colectomy (also known as proctocolectomy; "procto" from the Latin word "proctum," which means rectum) is removal of the colon, including the rectum. To do this, the anus must also be removed. Proctectomy means removal of the rectum. Another technical term for this is abdominoperineal resection, indicating that it is really two operations combined into one. Incisions must be made in both the abdomen and the perineum (the area between the anus and genitals).

Subtotal colectomy means removing all of the colon except the rectum. In the following pages, I use the term "near-total colectomy," which means removing all of the colon and most of the rectum. It is not a standard term, but is useful in explaining and understanding some of the operations done for IBD.

The suffix "ostomy" refers to a surgically created connection between a hollow organ and the skin, or between two hollow organs. "Resect" means cut out. "Anastomosis" refers to a surgically created connection. An ileostomy is an opening of the ileum out to the skin; a colostomy is the same thing using the colon. The plastic bag that fits over the opening at the skin, or stoma (meaning "mouth"), is called an "appliance."

The appliance is attached to a plastic ring that is kept in position on the abdominal wall by an adhesive paste. All ostomies, with one exception (see Kock ileostomy on page 119), require the wearing of an appliance.

Surgery for Ulcerative Colitis

About a third of all people with ulcerative colitis will undergo removal of the colon during their lifetime. This is for one of two main reasons: because medical therapy has failed to control the disease adequately; or because precancerous changes, or actual cancer, have been found in the colon. The best way to understand the various operations for ulcerative colitis is to review the history of surgery for this disease.

The 1930s and 1940s: Subtotal Colectomy, Ileostomy and Mucous Fistula of the Rectum

In the 1930s and 1940s, the favored operation for colitis was a subtotal colectomy with an ileostomy and a mucous fistula of the rectum. The rectum was not attached to the ileum, so the stool came out via the ileostomy.

The rectum was often severely inflamed in people having this surgery, and if the surgeon tried simply to sew up the top of the rectum, the stitches would often not hold and the contents of the rectum would leak into the abdomen — a dangerous complication. Surgeons figured out that if they brought the top of the rectum out to the skin, much like an ileostomy but smaller, such complications could be avoided. Mucous fistula of the rectum is the name for this procedure. As a result of improved surgical techniques, far fewer people have a mucous fistula of the rectum these days. Your surgeon will either remove the rectum during the initial operation or will leave the rectum in place but just close it at the top, with stitches or with staples.

MAKING AN ILEOSTOMY

When ileostomies were first done, the serosa of the ileum was simply sewn to the skin. (The serosa is the outer lining of the intestine and is much like the tough casing around a hot dog or a sausage.) This was easy to do, but unfortunately it did not work very well, because the outlet had a tendency to gradually become narrow in most cases. Patients would frequently develop obstruction at the ileostomy and have to be operated on again, often more than once.

The 1950s: The Brooke Ileostomy

In 1952, a British surgeon named Bryan Brooke solved the problem of ileostomy obstructions, by devising what has become known as the Brooke ileostomy. He figured that if the end of the ileum was folded over (much the way the end of a sleeve is folded over) and then attached to the skin, this would usually stop the ileostomy opening from shrinking and narrowing. He was right, and the success rate for ileostomies improved dramatically. In fact, this operation has stood the test of time and is still the standard technique for creating an ileostomy.

PROBLEMS ASSOCIATED WITH BROOKE ILEOSTOMIES

Although the majority of Brooke ileostomies are trouble-free, about 25 percent of patients will have problems. There is obviously a need for a psychological adjustment; this is frequently a major social issue

Brooke Ileostomy and Mucous Fistula of the Rectum

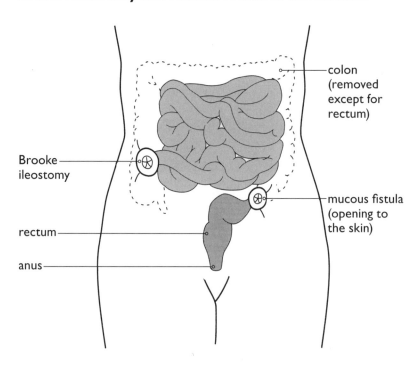

in school-age and unmarried people. In terms of physical activity, the only restriction relates to deep sea diving — you are not allowed to go down more than 110 feet (33 meters). Structural abnormalities can occur in and around the ileostomy, often needing surgical repair. Some people develop skin reactions to the stool, the appliance or the adhesives. Infection with a fungus is fairly common if the skin becomes raw, but this can be easily treated with an antifungal ointment. Leakage and odor are also possibilities that create concern. These problems can usually be treated by enterostomal therapists, nurses specializing in teaching patients about ostomies of various kinds. They are also specialists in solving various mechanical problems and skin irritation related to ostomies.

Many people with ileostomies must avoid high-roughage foods such as popcorn, nuts, sprouts, oranges and grapefruit or they may experience episodes of crampy abdominal pain, due to temporary blockage. As well, people with ileostomies need to pay attention to their fluid intake. Because output from the ileostomy contains more water than normal stool, not taking in enough fluids will result in less urine and an increased risk of kidney stones. You should always maintain a higher-than-normal fluid and salt intake and be particularly careful to avoid becoming dehydrated if diarrhea occurs for any reason, or if you develop fever, which causes more water to be lost as sweat. See Chapter 12 for more information.

The 1960s: The Kock Pouch (Kock Ileostomy, Continent Ileostomy)

In the late 1960s, a Swedish surgeon named Nils Kock came up with the idea of a continent ileostomy. "Continent" means that the patient controls the emptying of the ileostomy. (We don't refer to a Brooke ileostomy as an "incontinent ileostomy" — meaning the patient has no control over the emptying — but that's really what it is.)

Kock devised the ileal pouch or reservoir, which he constructed by sewing together two sections of ileum, each about 6 inches (15 centimeters) long. He determined that such a pouch would need a capacity of about 0.5 liter to act like a rectum and adequately store stool.

Kock then also devised the nipple valve. This uses the end of the ileum to create an ileostomy that acts like a one-way valve, preventing stool from coming out of the ileum on its own. To empty the pouch

A Kock Pouch and Ileostomy and Drainage of the Pouch

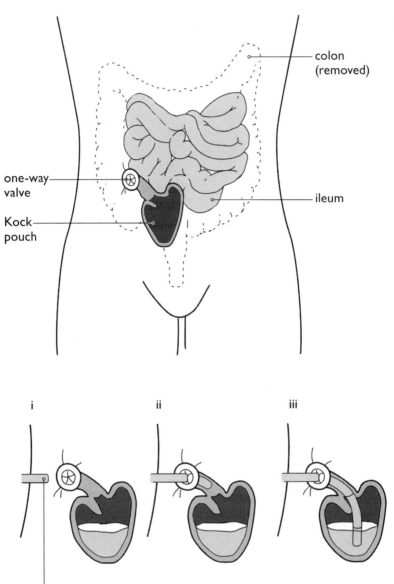

drainage tube is inserted by patient

or reservoir, you insert a tube through the nipple valve into the pouch and lean forward, and the reservoir empties through the tube into the toilet. You then pull the tube out, clean it and put it away for next time. Individuals having this surgery have a total proctocolectomy at the same time, removing the colon and rectum. When Kock first introduced this operation, it was a major step forward. However, it has been used much less since the introduction of the pelvic pouch procedure (see below). In fact, there are now only a few surgeons in North America who can perform this operation.

PROBLEMS ASSOCIATED WITH THE KOCK POUCH
Relatively few problems occur with the Kock procedure. The major problem is maintaining the valve in the proper position. In the early years (1970s and 1980s), the failure rate was 25 to 40 percent, defined as loss of continence. The valve can leak enough to require wearing an appliance (ostomy bag). In this case, a second operation must be done to correct the valve's function. The surgical term for this is "revision" of the valve, and two or three revisions of the valve may be necessary. Such operations are minor, but they still require a general anesthetic. Dr. Barnett, an American surgeon, designed a modification of the Kock valve, and claimed better results. (Visit www.kockpouch.com for more details.)

Inflammation of the inner lining of the pouch, known simply as pouchitis, is another common problem, and discussed in more detail later in this chapter. About one-third of continent ileostomy patients will have at least one episode of pouchitis within the first 5 years after surgery, compared to half of those people with a pelvic pouch.

WHY IS THIS OPERATION USED FOR ULCERATIVE COLITIS
BUT NOT USUALLY FOR CROHN'S DISEASE?
Because construction of the pouch requires about 1 foot (30 centimeters) of ileum, this operation is not done on people known to have small bowel Crohn's disease prior to surgery. The reason is that if Crohn's disease occurs in part of the pouch and you require surgical removal of the diseased area, then the whole pouch will have to be removed, even if the rest of it is normal. Neither doctors nor their patients like to give up any normal small bowel in Crohn's disease. However, this operation is an option in selected patients with Crohn's confined to the colon.

CARE OF THE KOCK ILEOSTOMY

If you have a properly functioning Kock pouch and nipple valve, you will experience little inconvenience. Many people wear a small dressing over the ileostomy to absorb the minor amount of mucus and other intestinal fluids produced locally by the mucosa (inner lining). There are no absolute dietary restrictions, but some individuals have difficulty with indigestibles such as seeds, apple skins and celery fibers. After you have fully recovered from surgery, there are no restrictions on activity. And there are no special problems associated with pregnancy.

If you have a Kock pouch with a continent ileostomy and are troubled by frequent pouchitis or repeated difficulties with a leaky valve, you can have surgery to change to a Brooke ileostomy. This happens to about one-third of people with a continent ileostomy.

The Present: The Pelvic Pouch with Ileo-Anal Anastomosis

It didn't take long for surgeons to realize that Kock's idea could be modified to create a pouch in the pelvis with the end of the ileum attached to the anus to allow "normal" bowel movements. This "pelvic pouch with ileo-anal anastomosis" operation was introduced in the late 1970s and has become the procedure of choice for most patients undergoing surgery for ulcerative colitis, and for selected people with Crohn's colitis. Because this surgery removes the rectum but still avoids a permanent stoma, it has also been called a "restorative proctocolectomy," meaning that it restores (relatively) normal bowel function.

However, the operation is generally not offered to people older than 65, as the anal sphincter muscle in older people tends to be weaker, and these individuals are much more likely to be troubled by incontinence of stool. People who have this operation at a younger age seem able to adapt better. For older patients, the best operation for ulcerative colitis is usually a total proctocolectomy and Brooke ileostomy, which requires wearing an appliance. If such a patient is ill or malnourished, or is unwell because of other medical conditions, the best operation is a subtotal colectomy with a Brooke ileostomy and a remaining, but disconnected, rectum. The rectum may be removed at a later date. In some IBD centers, age alone is not reason enough to refuse someone a pelvic-pouch operation.

HOW IS THE PELVIC-POUCH OPERATION DONE?

The pelvic-pouch operation can be done as a three-stage, two-stage or one-stage procedure. When a surgeon tells you that you are going to have a three-stage operation, you should understand that this means you are going to have three operations. It's easy to understand why surgeons prefer to say a "three-stage operation" — many people would be frightened to death if they had to think about having three operations for one problem. Nevertheless, that is actually what happens.

THE THREE-STAGE PROCEDURE

If someone with ulcerative colitis is ill and requires surgery, it will most likely be a three-stage procedure. In the first stage, you will have a subtotal colectomy, construction of a Brooke ileostomy and either a mucous fistula of the rectum or a simple closure of the top of the rectum, without a mucous fistula. Someone in this situation will almost certainly be on steroids, and likely other medications as well. Following the operation, you will be allowed to recover, and your medications will be tapered off and stopped. After an interval of 3 to 6 months, the second stage will be done. Some people are anxious to get rid of the ileostomy (and the appliance) as soon as possible. But results following the second stage are generally better if you have regained full health and are off most or all medications, especially steroids.

In the second stage, most of the rectum will be removed, and the pelvic pouch will be constructed and connected. Strictly speaking, the ileum is not connected directly to the anus. The surgeon has to leave a very short segment of the bottom of the rectum for the end of the ileum to be attached to. In the early days of this operation, some surgeons removed the bit of mucosa left in this segment to totally eliminate the colitis, but it is now left in to reduce the risk of incontinence.

An ileostomy will again be created. The Brooke ileostomy is also known as an end ileostomy because it is made by bringing the end of the ileum out through the abdominal wall. When the pelvic pouch is created, the end of the ileum is connected to the beginning of the anus. The ileostomy created during this second operation is known as a loop ileostomy. With this ileostomy, a hole is made in the side of the ileum, and that is attached to the skin. The purpose of the loop ileostomy, which is temporary, is to divert stool before it gets down to the pouch and ileo-anal anastomosis. The reason is to create the best possible conditions for this complex surgery to heal. This process of healing generally takes 2 to 3 months.

You will then return for the third stage of the procedure. This is a relatively minor operation, but it still requires a general anesthetic. Here the loop ileostomy is closed so that you can begin having bowel movements "the normal way." If you are not particularly ill, this three-stage operation can be combined into two stages. In the first stage, you will have a near-total colectomy, and the pelvic pouch, the ileo-anal anastomosis and the loop ileostomy will be created. About 3 months later, the loop ileostomy will be closed.

At the beginning of the 1990s, IBD surgeons began experimenting with doing the entire operation in one stage. While this is appealing, more patients have postsurgical complications than those with the temporary loop ileostomy, so the one-stage procedure is done only in carefully selected individuals.

SIDE EFFECTS AND COMPLICATIONS OF PELVIC-POUCH SURGERY
This surgery involves the risk of several side effects and complications.

Frequent or urgent bowel movements, or both. Pelvic-pouch surgery allows you a return to health, but many people still have an average of 4 to 8 semiformed bowel movements a day and 1 movement per night. This varies considerably — some people have 10 to 12 per 24 hours, or even more. You may be much better off taking regular doses of loperamide, diphenoxylate or codeine (see Chapter 6), with supplemental doses as necessary. Even without antidiarrheal drugs, urgency is not a problem for most patients.

Incontinence. If someone with a pelvic pouch has frequent, unpredictable bowel movements, with episodes of incontinence, little has been achieved, even though the colitis is cured. In the first 6 months or so after closure of the loop ileostomy, many people have quite frequent stools and some degree of urgency. A small number are troubled by incontinence during the day. A somewhat larger number are troubled by incontinence that occurs only at night. The reason for this difference is that everyone passes gas from the rectum while asleep. If there is less-than-normal sensitivity in the anal canal, and particularly if

Pelvic Pouch Procedure with Ileo-Anal Anastomosis

First stage

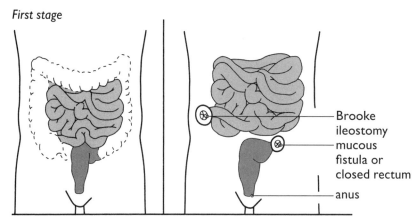

Brooke
ileostomy

mucous
fistula or
closed rectum

anus

Second stage

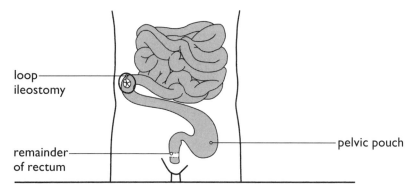

loop
ileostomy

remainder
of rectum

pelvic pouch

Third stage

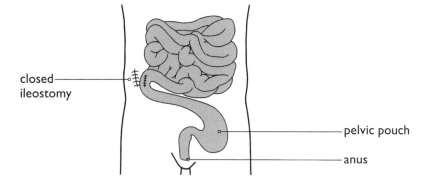

closed
ileostomy

pelvic pouch

anus

loose stool is present, the gas may be accompanied by a small amount of fluid without you being aware of it. Many people wear a pad at night; only a few need to wear one during the day. Some people have more than a little incontinence of stool, and this is a major problem.

Be patient. Fortunately, a significant degree of adaptation occurs during the first 3 to 6 months following the operation. The pouch gets larger and "learns" to store stool, acting like a rectum. As this happens, the daily number of trips to the bathroom usually decreases, and incontinence also decreases. Still, like many people, you may continue to wear a pad at night for psychological comfort, even after the incontinence is gone.

If incontinence remains a major problem, there is usually little choice but to give up the pelvic pouch. You can then have a Kock ileostomy (if you have access to a surgeon who can do it), or, to have the best chance of not needing any further surgery, you can have a Brooke ileostomy. Aside from the need for psychological adjustment to the idea of a permanent stoma, the main disadvantage of the conversion to a Brooke ileostomy is that you have to lose the whole pouch, about 18 inches (45 centimeters) of healthy ileum, as the pouch cannot be taken apart.

Pouchitis. Whether you have a Kock pouch higher up in the abdomen in combination with a continent ileostomy or a pelvic pouch with an ileo-anal anastomosis, inflammation of the pouch is a common prob-

---

Who Can Have a Kock Pouch and Ileostomy?
(if you have access to a surgeon who can do this operation)
The Kock (continent) ileostomy is an alternative to the Brooke ileostomy for certain colitis patients in the following groups:
- those with a Brooke ileostomy who have had a total proctocolectomy and who wish to avoid wearing an appliance;
- those who need a colectomy but are not candidates for a pelvic pouch, usually because of poor anal-sphincter function;
- those who prefer a continent ileostomy to a pelvic pouch with ileo-anal anastomosis — usually people who cannot make frequent trips to the bathroom because of their jobs;
- those who have had a failed ileo-anal anastomosis but still prefer continence to wearing an external appliance.

lem. Doctors seem to make up complicated-sounding names for many diseases, but this is a definite exception. The condition is simply called pouchitis. It is usually accompanied by loose stools, a need to empty the pouch more frequently and, sometimes, abdominal pain. Blood may be present in the stool. Most cases respond well to antibiotics; both ciprofloxacin and metronidazole are commonly used, alone or combined. Budesonide enemas are also effective in some cases. Studies have shown that pouchitis can often be prevented from coming back by using the probiotic product VSL-3 (see Chapter 5). Starting VSL-3 immediately after closure of a loop ileostomy may reduce the risk of developing pouchitis. The cause of pouchitis is unknown. Persistent pouchitis raises the possibility of Crohn's disease.

Sexual dysfunction and fertility. Most people report that sexual function is unchanged or improved following surgery. Improvement usually reflects better general health. However, of men having this surgery, 1 to 2 percent become impotent or are unable to reach orgasm after surgery; about 4 percent experience retrograde ejaculation, which means that the semen goes into the bladder instead of coming out of the penis. In women, frequency of intercourse and ability to reach orgasm tend to increase after surgery, and painful intercourse decreases.

Female fertility rates in ulcerative colitis are typically normal up to the time of surgery. Female fertility after the pelvic-pouch operation is reduced. Dense scar tissue formation involving the ovaries or Fallopian tubes, or both, may be the reason. In vitro fertilization (IVF) is an option for those women who are unable to conceive within a reasonable time after full recovery from surgery.

Narrowing of the anastomosis. Some people make more scar tissue than others. Because the scar tissue encircles a tube (the anal canal), its inevitable shrinkage during healing may produce narrowing. In about 5 percent of patients undergoing ileo-anal anastomosis, the narrowing causes difficulty passing stool; this is called a stricture and develops at the site of the anastomosis. This can usually be treated by dilatation (stretching), which is a simple procedure done with a local anesthetic or sedative, or both, but usually not requiring a general anesthetic.

Postoperative leak. Postoperative leaks happen occasionally with any type of bowel surgery and do not reflect badly on the surgeon. If a leak occurs, an abscess (boil) is likely to form next to the anastomosis. This will result in pain in the pelvis or around the anus, and fever. The abscess will generally require drainage, either by inserting a very fine needle into it to extract the pus or by making a small cut into the abscess with a scalpel so the pus can drain on its own. Sometimes infection due to a leak will clear up simply with antibiotic therapy. Repeated abscess formation suggests Crohn's disease. Even if that is not the cause, a loop ileostomy may have to be recreated to allow healing.

Inflammation at the anastomosis (known as cuffitis). Because most people are left with a tiny piece (like a cuff) of rectal lining, it is possible to have persistent or recurrent colitis in this area. About 10 percent of people will have symptoms, such as urgency or bleeding. Treatment with suppositories (5-ASA or hydrocortisone) is usually effective.

Cancer. Cancer of the colon occurs more commonly in people with colitis than it does in the general population. When the whole colon is removed (total proctocolectomy), the risk is removed. When a person undergoes a pouch procedure with an ileo-anal anastomosis, a tiny cuff of colon (the last bit of the rectum) is usually left in, to provide better continence. Even if the surgeon peels off whatever can be seen of the inner lining of the colon (not usually done), it is always possible that a few microscopic glands will be left behind. These glands could at some point give rise to a cancer. With the current practice of leaving the very small amount of mucosa intact, the risk is slightly greater, but overall it is still extremely low.

PELVIC-POUCH PROCEDURE FOR THOSE WITH INDETERMINATE COLITIS

We are unable to distinguish ulcerative colitis from Crohn's disease in about 10 percent of patients. In most IBD centers, if surgery is needed, such patients are given the benefit of the doubt and are offered a pelvic-pouch procedure with ileo-anal anastomosis. However, they should understand that the chances that this operation will fail are higher than they are for people with clear-cut ulcerative colitis. Still, the chances of success are reasonably good. If the problem is in fact ulcerative colitis, the failure rate will be no more than usual. If it is Crohn's disease, about 65 percent of people will be disease-free 10 years later.

Surgery for Crohn's Disease

Surgery for ulcerative colitis involves removing most or all of the colon. Surgery for Crohn's disease depends on where in the GI tract the disease occurs.

People with Crohn's disease require surgery for one of three main reasons: the failure of medical therapy to control the disease adequately, chronic or frequently recurring obstructions, and abscesses with or without fistulas (abnormal channels).

The decision that surgery is needed because medical therapy has failed to control the disease adequately should be made jointly by the gastroenterologist, the surgeon and the patient (or patient's parents). The criteria may be different for different people.

Obstructions

You can think of the normal intestine as an elastic band. It has a thin wall; the opening is large in relation to the thickness of the wall, and it is able to stretch easily. When Crohn's disease occurs in the intestine, the wall becomes swollen. It swells outward, but it also swells inward. Now the intestine is more like a tire. It is still somewhat stretchy, but the wall is thicker and stiffer and the channel is much narrower.

Thickening of Intestinal Wall

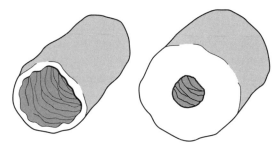

During an acute obstruction, the swelling increases even more. The wall swells outward more (which is not a problem), but it also swells inward more. The intestinal channel does not have to be completely blocked to act blocked. If someone with acute small bowel obstruction goes on a clear-fluid diet or takes prednisone, the swelling will almost always decrease and the obstruction will get better, usually within 48 hours.

If the person begins to have frequently recurring obstructions or has some symptoms of obstruction all the time (nausea, bloating and crampy abdominal pain soon after every meal), the narrowing of the intestine is likely due not only to swelling but also to scarring. Steroids, a biological or an enteral (sterilized liquid) diet should reduce the swelling. But when the narrowing is due mainly to scarring, no drug or diet treatment will relieve the problem for long, if at all.

An area of scarring may be dilated with an inflatable balloon passed through an endoscope. Improvements in equipment have raised the success rate in experienced hands to as high as 75 percent; relief of obstructive symptoms can last weeks, months or years. However, the area has to be accessible to an endoscope. If a balloon dilation is not possible, then an operation is necessary.

There are two types of surgery for small bowel Crohn's disease: strictureplasty and resection. The term "strictureplasty" comes from "stricture," meaning narrowing, and "plasty," meaning shaping something through the use of surgery. You can think of the procedure as plastic surgery on the intestine. Resection means removing something by cutting it out.

The idea in strictureplasty is to take a narrowed area of intestine and make it wider. People with Crohn's disease of the small bowel who should be considered for this type of surgery fall into two groups: those who have had a previous resection and need another operation, and those who need surgery and have never had it before but have very extensive disease. Some people undergoing strictureplasty also require resection of additional segments of diseased intestine that are not suitable for strictureplasty.

Although it is medically desirable to be on at least one of the drugs that can heal the residual disease *and* maintain remission, many people who undergo strictureplasty are able to stop taking most of their medications, eat normally and gain weight. In long-term follow-up, the majority of strictures that are opened in this way remain open.

Strictureplasty

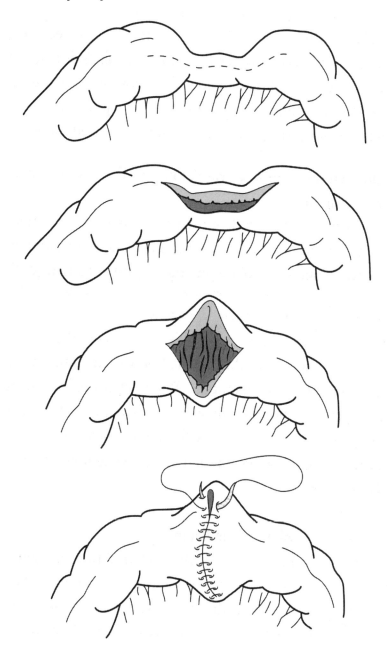

When people who have had strictureplasty require surgery for obstruction again, it is usually due to the formation of new strictures.

What is interesting about this surgery is that the Crohn's disease in the area of the operated-on stricture improves considerably after the operation. When strictureplasty patients are operated upon for some other reason, the areas of strictureplasty usually appear much less inflamed than before the strictureplasty. We can conclude that, while the disease itself causes the narrowing, the narrowing somehow makes the disease worse.

Surgery for Crohn's of the Ileum

Although Crohn's disease is often referred to as a segmental or patchy disease, in most people the disease occurs at the end of the ileum, with or without involving the cecum (the beginning of the colon, where the appendix is). When such people require surgery for the first time, they usually have a resection of the area of the disease with anastomosis (connection) of the new end of the ileum (referred to as the neo-terminal ileum) to the ascending colon in one of two ways.

Some people having a resection have one or more fistulas from the area of disease to another part of the intestine that is not affected by Crohn's disease. The surgeon may have to remove a little piece of intestine where the fistula runs in. If you have such a fistula and it leads to the last 1 to 2 feet (30 or 60 centimeters) of the colon, you may need a temporary stoma to divert the stool away from the site of the repaired fistula, allowing the colon to rest and heal properly. In a minor operation, the stoma will be closed 1 to 2 months later.

Common Side Effects of Resection of the End of the Ileum

Removing the end of the ileum is not without consequences. The major ones are discussed below.

Diarrhea due to loss of the ileocecal valve. The ileocecal valve allows liquid intestinal contents to be discharged into the colon in a controlled, intermittent fashion. Surgical removal can lead to diarrhea. This effect is almost always temporary.

Bile-salt diarrhea. Normally, 90 to 99 percent of bile salts reaching the ileum are recycled back to the liver and reused. The remaining

1 to 10 percent is lost into the colon. When even a bit of ileum is removed, the amount lost each day into the colon is increased. Certain bile salts have a laxative-like effect on the colon, and the colon loses salt and water instead of absorbing them as it is supposed to. The result is diarrhea. Fortunately, bile-salt diarrhea is usually easy to control with drugs (see Chapter 6).

Decreased fat digestion and absorption. When you undergo resection of more than about 3 feet (1 meter) of the end of the ileum, two things happen. First, the liver is unable to maintain a normal level of bile salts in the intestine to digest fat. Second, large resections such as this interfere with absorption of the fat that *is* digested because fat requires the greatest length of intestine for its absorption.

If cholestyramine is being used to treat bile-salt diarrhea, that drug will further reduce the quantity of available bile salts, and this will further interfere with fat digestion and, indirectly, with fat absorption. Unabsorbed fat is broken down by bacteria in the colon, producing chemicals that have a laxative effect, possibly aggravating the diarrhea. Fortunately, a relatively small number of patients end up having more than 3 feet (about 1 meter) of ileum removed, even when they require a second or third resection.

Decreased vitamin B12 absorption. Another function of the ileum is to absorb vitamin B12. If a portion of your ileum is removed, you may have subnormal vitamin B12 absorption. If less than 8 inches (20 centimeters) of your ileum was removed, you should still have normal vitamin B12 absorption. If you have had removal of 8 to 24 inches (20 to 60 centimeters) of ileum, your B12 absorption may or may not be adequate. In the past, a Schilling test was done a few months after the resection to determine whether B12 absorption was normal. Although the test has no risks and is very accurate, it is much less available than it used to be. If more than 2 feet (60 centimeters) of your ileum has been removed, B12 absorption will *not* be normal, and there's no point to doing a Schilling test.

For the Schilling test, you are given an injection of B12 and then asked to drink a fluid containing a tracer amount of radioactive B12 (don't worry, there's no danger to you). Then you collect your urine for 2 days — in a separate container for each day — and the radio-

Surgery for the Most Common Form of Crohn's Disease

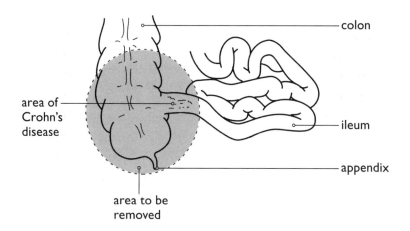

colon

area of
Crohn's
disease

ileum

appendix

area to be
removed

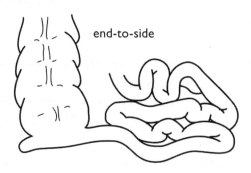

end-to-side

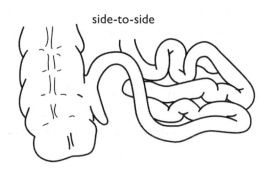

side-to-side

activity is measured to indicate the amount of B12 that your body absorbed. But if your doctor can't arrange a Schilling test or feels that it is unnecessary, then you should be told whether you need supplementary B12.

Some doctors simply put their patients on B12 shots after resection of a piece of ileum. However, these injections are once a month — forever. Fortunately, research has shown that most of such patients can still absorb *oral* B12, provided they take enough. Our bodies need 1 to 2 micrograms a day. The minimum effective oral dose for people with ileal resection is 1,000 micrograms per day. This means taking a pill every day, but there's no need for injections. Your doctor should measure your blood level once or twice a year to make sure you're taking enough. Vitamin B12 itself has no side effects, but occasionally people will experience some kind of side effect from the nonmedicinal ingredients in the tablets. If you do not go on supplemental B12, your blood level of B12 should be measured once or twice a year. However, don't be lulled by one or two normal results. The body can have several years' worth of B12 stored up in the liver, but the supply will eventually run out. In some countries, you can get a B12 product in the form of a nose spray. You may prefer this, but it is expensive and must be used twice a week. Whatever you do, remember that a lack of vitamin B12 can cause brain damage, so don't forget about it!

Short Bowel Syndrome

As noted, many people with small bowel Crohn's disease require more than one operation. A small number will end up with not enough bowel surface area to allow normal digestion and absorption of nutrients. This is known as short bowel syndrome. Some of these people can cope by having a restricted diet and using specialized products such as MCT oil; some will need home TPN (see Chapter 5). *Some* people with short bowel syndrome will be able to nourish themselves adequately without restrictions or supplements but will not be able to maintain normal water balance — they usually get the extra water they need by receiving intravenous fluid every night, while they are asleep.

Surgery for Crohn's Disease of the Jejunum

Most jejunal disease is treated by resection, but some people undergo strictureplasty. The ileum is able to compensate completely for the loss of the jejunum, even with extensive resections, so side effects of jejunal resection are uncommon.

Surgery for Crohn's Disease of the Duodenum

A few people develop narrowing of the lumen (channel) in the duodenum, so that food cannot pass. Resection or strictureplasty surgery is technically difficult because of the duodenum's anatomic location, but strictureplasty is possible in some cases. When it isn't, a bypass operation called a gastrojejunostomy is done. In this operation, a loop of upper jejunum is surgically attached (anastomosed) to the stomach. Several side effects may occur, a discussion of which is beyond the scope of this book.

Surgery for Crohn's Disease of the Stomach

People with Crohn's of the stomach rarely require surgery. If they do, it is mainly because of narrowing and obstruction of the lower third of the stomach. The usual operation is a gastrojejunostomy, as described above.

Surgery for Crohn's Disease of the Esophagus

Esophageal Crohn's disease is rare. Part or all of the esophagus (swallowing tube) can be removed, if necessary. Some surgeons simply pull the stomach up into the chest and connect it to the remaining esophagus. Others use a section of the patient's jejunum or colon to bridge the gap.

Surgery for Crohn's Disease of the Colon (Crohn's Colitis)

Surgery for Crohn's disease of the colon varies according to how much of the colon is involved, how severe the disease is, what the surgeon and gastroenterologist advise and what the patient or patient's family wants. The common reasons for surgery for Crohn's colitis are the same as for Crohn's disease in general — failure of medical therapy to control the disease, abscesses with or without fistulas, obstructions —and for cancer.

Side Effects of Surgery for Crohn's Colitis

After small segments of the colon are surgically removed, bowel habits should generally be normal. But since the function of the colon is to remove water from the stool, the more colon that is lost, the more likely it is that you will have diarrhea. This can often be controlled with antidiarrheal drugs. That being said, many people have remarkably normal bowel habits even if they are left with only about 1 foot (30 centimeters) of colon above the rectum (ileo-sigmoid anastomosis).

Side Effects of Ostomies with the Rectum or Rectum and More of the Colon Left in Place

As we learned in Chapter 1, most of the waste material in the colon consists of mucus, living and dead bacteria, and dead lining cells of the bowel. Even if the rectum is disconnected, it continues to produce mucus, provide a home for bacteria and shed its lining regularly. In other words, it continues to make stool.

Although there is no food residue, the stool that is made accumulates and must be emptied every so often. Some people make more; others make less. But everyone who has a disconnected rectum will continue to have the urge to have a bowel movement in the normal way every so often. Some patients, particularly those who have not been warned, are confused when they get the urge to go to the toilet. "I must be going crazy," you may think. "My rectum is disconnected from my intestines, but I still feel I have to have a bowel movement!" Of course you're not crazy; you are simply getting the urge to pass the nonfood portion of the stool.

You shouldn't resist the urge. If you do, the stool will accumulate. Just like normal stool that is held in, it will get drier and drier and harder and harder. It will accumulate until the rectum fills up. When that happens, you will generally start to get increasing pressure and discomfort in the pelvic region. Sooner or later you'll see a doctor, who will examine you and find that the rectum is full. Some patients find it necessary to give themselves a small enema every so often.

Diversion Colitis

Doctors often refer to the creation of either an ileostomy or a colostomy as a "diverting" procedure. We say that the "fecal stream" has been diverted — similar to creating a detour on a road. The Crohn's

Surgery for Crohn's Colitis

Location of Disease	Possible Operations	Advantages	Disadvantages
Most or all of colon (including rectum)	Total proctococlectomy and Brooke ileostomy	Lowest chance of recurrence	Perineal incision that may not heal completely Need appliance
	Subtotal colectomy, Brooke ileostomy, oversewn rectum	No perineal incision	Risk of persistent or recurrent disease in rectum Access to rectal cancer checkup may be difficult Need appliance
Most or all of colon, but normal rectum	Total proctocolectomy and Brooke ileostomy	Lowest chance of recurrence	Perineal incision Need appliance
	Subtotal colectomy, Brooke ileostomy, oversewn rectum	No perineal incision	Risk of persistent or recurrent disease in rectum Need appliance Access to rectal cancer checkup may be difficult
	Subtotal colectomy, and ileorectal anastomosis	No perineal incision No need for appliance	Highest chance of recurrent disease in ileum or rectum Need for cancer surveillance of rectum Frequent bowel movements ☛

Location of Disease	Possible Operations	Advantages	Disadvantages
Short segment (excluding rectum)	Segmental resection	Low chance of diarrhea Simple operation	High chance of recurrent disease
Rectum only	Colostomy only	Simple operation	Possible or persistent or or recurrent rectal or perianal disease Need for appliance
	Colostomy and proctectomy	Better chance of prolonged relief of symptons	Perineal incision Need for appliance
Ileum and colon	Selective, if symptoms are distinctively ileum or colon	Conserves bowel (fewer side effects)	Higher recurrence rate

disease that is downstream of the diversion usually heals. However, in many people, a different type of inflammation develops in whatever part of the colon is downstream. This inflammation is called diversion colitis.

In the 1980s, researchers discovered that diversion colitis occurs because colonic lining cells require substances known as short-chain fatty acids to be healthy. Short-chain fatty acids are normally produced by the colonic bacteria that break down complex carbohydrate residue (i.e., undigested fiber) from our diet. The researchers showed that giving short-chain fatty acid enemas to such people could heal this form of colitis. They also showed that closing the ostomy and restoring the continuity of the bowel achieve the same thing.

With the colonoscope and under the microscope, diversion colitis can look like ulcerative colitis, Crohn's colitis or neither. Furthermore, this kind of colitis can lead to the formation of strictures. If a person has had a diverting operation, and the surgeon is planning to reconnect the bowel, it is important to do a colonoscopy or an imaging study, such as a CT scan, or both, and examine the disconnected part of the colon. If there are strictures, they will probably have to be resected (cut out) at the time of surgery. If the diversion colitis is severe, it may be worthwhile to treat the patient with short-chain fatty acid enemas for a couple of weeks prior to surgery. If the diversion colitis is mild, nothing needs to be done. Other than the usual mechanical risk of having an enema, there are no side effects with this treatment.

No commercial short-chain fatty acid product exists. It is usually manufactured by hospital pharmacies at the request of a gastroenterologist. Because this is not a marketed product, most drug plans do not pay for it. There is no oral form.

Lastly, if there is no intent to reconnect the bowel, it's important for you and your doctor to remember that you have a portion of your colon there, as it should be included in any cancer surveillance program (see Chapter 10).

Recurring Crohn's Disease after Surgery

The chance of Crohn's disease coming back after surgery is highest if you have combined small bowel and colon disease, slightly lower if you have pure small bowel disease and lowest if you have pure colon disease, provided you have had all of the colon removed, or all of the colon except for the rectum. Just to make things more confusing, there are three kinds of recurrence referred to in the medical literature. One kind is *endoscopic recurrence* — that is, recurrent disease that is found by examining your bowel with a scope. European researchers have demonstrated that many people undergoing small bowel resection have evidence of new disease in the ileum visible with the colonoscope within 12 weeks of surgery; however, the vast majority of these patients will not have symptoms at that time. *Clinical recurrence* is what is of concern to most patients — a return of symptoms and signs of the disease. *Surgical recurrence* is defined as the need for further surgery. Despite numerous studies, we have little knowledge about the factors that influence clinically recurrent Crohn's disease. We do know that smoking increases the risk and stopping smoking decreases it.

For individuals with pure small bowel disease or those with combined small and large bowel disease, most recurrences will be in the ileum, starting from the anastomosis (connection) and extending upward. Why it is much less common for the disease to recur downstream from the anastomosis is just one more mystery of Crohn's disease. The symptoms, signs and extent of disease prior to surgery cannot be used to predict the symptoms, signs and extent when the disease comes back.

Current figures indicate that 70 to 90 percent of people will have endoscopic recurrence within 1 year after small bowel resection, although the majority of them will not have any clinical signs or symptoms of the disease. About 15 percent to 25 percent of patients with small bowel disease (with or without colonic disease) will have symptoms (clinical recurrence) of the disease within 2 years of surgery, 30 to 50 percent within about 5 years and about 70 percent within 10 years. It is believed that if people lived long enough, the recurrence rate of small bowel Crohn's would be 100 percent.

For disease of the colon, the situation is not so clear. If a short segment of diseased colon is removed, there is probably a 75 percent chance of developing further disease. But if the entire colon plus rectum is removed, some IBD centers suggest that the recurrence rate in the ileum will be as low as 10 percent, while other equally authoritative centers suggest that the risk is as high as 40 percent. There is also a higher risk of recurrent Crohn's disease in the ileum in people who undergo subtotal colectomy and ileo-rectal anastomosis than in those with subtotal colectomy and ileostomy. On the other hand, the chance that someone will need removal of the rectum (proctectomy) is higher in people who have had an ileostomy (60 percent in 10 years) than in those with an ileorectal anastomosis (20 percent). This is probably because those with an ileostomy are more likely to have had significant rectal disease before surgery.

Can Someone with Crohn's Disease Have a Pelvic-Pouch Operation?

Some doctors feel that this is an option for selected patients with Crohn's in the colon only. It seems important that such people have no history, past or present, of small bowel Crohn's, or of anal involvement.

One of the reasons the statistics on surgery for Crohn's colitis are so confusing is that far fewer patients require surgery compared with people who have Crohn's disease of the ileum, or of the ileum and colon. So in any given center for IBD there may not be enough patients to provide statistically meaningful numbers about the outcome of a particular operation.

Looking at Crohn's disease overall, without regard to where the disease occurs, various studies have suggested that the lifetime chance of needing *any* surgery (including small operations such as drainage of a perianal abscess) for Crohn's disease is about 70 percent. Until recently, the chance of needing a second operation after a first resection was 25 to 40 percent at 5 years, 30 to 60 percent at 10 years and 40 to 70 percent at 20 years. New evidence suggests that the addition of biological drugs will reduce these numbers.

Laparoscopic Surgery for Ulcerative Colitis and Crohn's Disease

Recent reports indicate that all standard operations for IBD can be performed using laparoscopic techniques. (See the sidebar "Laparoscopic Surgery" for more details.) However, the surgeon's prior experience with these techniques is important, particularly when dealing with ill patients or complications.

Just because an operation can be done this way doesn't mean it's the best way for everyone. Some complex cases are better managed with laparoscopic-assisted surgery; this means that one incision (and one scar) will be larger than the others, but not as large as the typical scar from open surgery. This technique is generally chosen to shorten the length of an operation. Other advantages of laparoscopic surgery

---

Laparoscopic Surgery

Laparoscopic surgery is popularly known as "keyhole surgery" because the surgeon gets into the patient's abdomen through a series of "keyhole" incisions — little cuts through the abdominal wall. Carbon dioxide gas (which is safe) is pumped into the abdomen to create some space between the organs, allowing the surgeon to see what he or she is doing. Various instruments are placed through these incisions, and an operation is performed with the aid of a television-video system.

include less pain after surgery, less time in the hospital and more rapid recovery. The cosmetic result — much smaller scars — is particularly valuable for children and young adults.

Small Bowel Transplantation

This form of treatment is technically challenging. While it is sometimes successful, its use is generally restricted to people who must come off home TPN because of advanced liver disease (in which case it is combined with a liver transplantation), recurrent blood clots in major veins or a lack of adequate veins for administration of the TPN because of previous clots or infection, or both, resulting in scarring and blockage of the veins.

Surgical Treatment for Abscesses and Fistulas

About 25 percent of people with Crohn's disease are troubled by perianal disease, which means disease around the anus. The problems that usually require surgery include abscesses (boils) and fistulas (see Chapter 9).

How Does an Abscess Form?

Abscesses and fistulas in Crohn's disease arise because of little breaks in the inner lining of the small or large intestine. These breaks allow germs (such as bacteria) that are normally present in the intestine to get into tissues such as the mesentery or the tissues around the rectum, where they shouldn't be. This is referred to as a confined perforation. The presence of the germs triggers a response by the body to an invading force: the body sends in white blood cells (the army) to attack the bacteria. The white cells kill some bacteria, and the bacteria kill some white cells. Initially, the white cells win. However, once the break in the lining lets germs exit from the small bowel or colon, it almost always stays open. Bacteria thus continue to enter the tissues, and this leads to a continuing infection, a continuing response by the body and a continuing presence of white blood cells. The result is the gradual accumulation of pus, which is a mixture of living and dead white cells and living and dead bacteria. A common example of pus in everyday life is the yellow or green stuff that comes out of your nose when you have a bad cold.

Initially with an abscess, you don't feel anything. But gradually the accumulating pus puts pressure on the adjacent tissues. Sooner or later, the infection results in swelling and pain, and possibly a fever as well.

How Is an Abscess Treated?

The treatment for a collection of pus is to drain it. Sometimes the body will cause the drainage to occur without a doctor having to do anything. Think of having an acne pimple on your forehead. As the pimple grows, it becomes more and more uncomfortable because the skin around the pimple is being stretched due to the pressure of the pus within it. Many people with a painful acne pimple will squeeze it because they know that this will pop a little hole in the surface of the skin, most of the pus will drain out and the pain will go away. A somewhat more pleasant way of accomplishing the same thing is to apply warm wet compresses to the area. This will soften the skin and make it easier for the pimple to spring a leak and drain itself. An abdominal or perianal abscess is really just like a giant pimple. If the abscess bulges toward the surface of the abdomen or buttock, it may drain spontaneously. If you soak the area (by taking sitz baths, if it is a perianal abscess) this will encourage drainage. The skin in the area of the abscess softens and the pressure inside the abscess may cause it to break open and drain. Unfortunately, an abscess must often become quite large before it bulges the surface of the skin, and this means that it can become quite painful.

Many people cannot tolerate the pain while waiting for an abscess to drain spontaneously. Indeed, *they should not wait* — occasionally, an abscess can make you quite ill. At a hospital or doctor's office the abscess can be drained by freezing the area and making a small hole with a scalpel or a needle through the skin directly into the abscess. If a perianal abscess is large, you may have to be taken to the operating room and given a general anesthetic so a surgeon can adequately drain it. Large abdominal abscesses are almost always easily drained with the aid of ultrasound or CT scan guidance.

Draining the abscess does not always end the problem in people with Crohn's disease. As mentioned above, in most cases, the little opening in the inner lining of the intestine that led to the abscess remains. Draining an abscess results in a connection between the inside of the intestine and the outside world via the skin. This connection is one example of a fistula.

How an Abscess Forms in Crohn's Disease

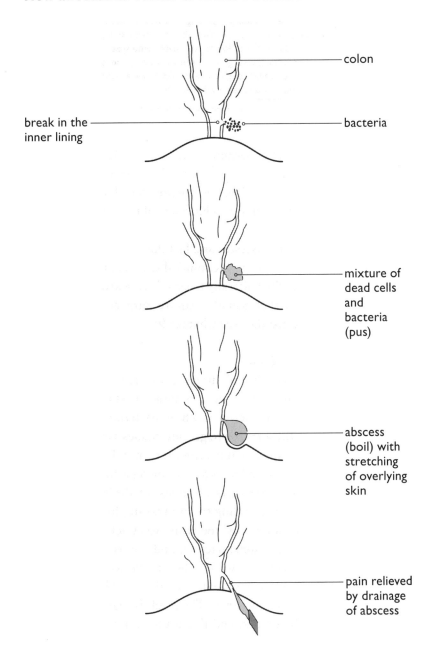

colon

break in the inner lining

bacteria

mixture of dead cells and bacteria (pus)

abscess (boil) with stretching of overlying skin

pain relieved by drainage of abscess

What is a Fistula?

A fistula is an abnormal connection between a hollow structure (such as the rectum) and the skin surface or between two hollow structures such as two loops of bowel, or bowel and bladder, or bowel and vagina. The path that the fistula follows is referred to as a "fistulous tract," and may be short or quite long.

Perianal Fistula

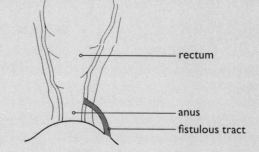

rectum

anus
fistulous tract

Recto-vaginal Fistula

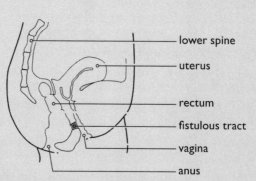

lower spine

uterus

rectum

fistulous tract

vagina

anus

Ileo-vesical (Ileum-to-bladder) Fistula

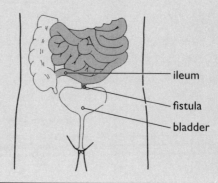

ileum

fistula

bladder

If a perianal abscess does not point toward the skin but points and presses instead on the patient's bladder, it may drain spontaneously into the bladder. This will solve the immediate problem of the abscess, but you'll be left with a fistula to the bladder that requires treatment. The same situation can occur if the abscess points toward and pushes on the vagina. If a fistula to the bladder, vagina or skin surface in a location other than the perineum is treated surgically, removal of the piece of intestine that is the source of the fistula is usually necessary. Some vaginal fistulas are not treated; if they are small, they may be just a minor nuisance. Some fistulas simply connect two segments of intestine; often nothing needs to be done about these either.

Sometimes multiple breaks in the lining occur close together. This may result in a large mass of inflamed tissue containing many little abscesses, called a phlegmon. Treatment for this condition is often surgical resection of the segment of intestine that is the source of infection, although some people will respond to antibiotics, which may be combined with a temporary enteral diet.

Treatment of a Chronic Abscess

Many people with perianal abscesses can be treated with sitz baths and antibiotics, but some need surgery. In some cases the surgeon must create a wedge-shaped opening into the abscess to clean it out thoroughly. Afterward, the wound cavity may be packed with gauze, which is usually changed daily. If this is not done, the wound usually closes over at the surface faster than it does deeper down, so that the abscess cavity remains and becomes filled with pus again. The packing keeps the skin wound open so that the wound heals from the bottom up (or, to put it another way, from the inside out).

If the procedure is totally successful, the area heals completely, leaving a scar. However, in most cases the patient is left with a fistulous tract, which is a narrow, straight, tube-like path from the inside of the bowel out to the skin, without an abscess cavity. Drainage is sometimes a relatively minor problem and some people tolerate it, rather than add or change drugs.

Use of Setons

Particularly if surgical treatment of a perianal fistula is going to be followed by anti-TNF therapy, it is important to try to make sure that

Fistula Tract with Chronic Abscess

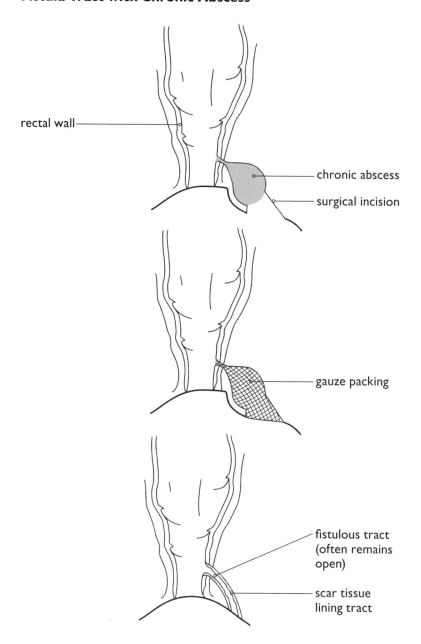

rectal wall

chronic abscess

surgical incision

gauze packing

fistulous tract
(often remains
open)

scar tissue
lining tract

Placement of Seton for Perianal Fistula

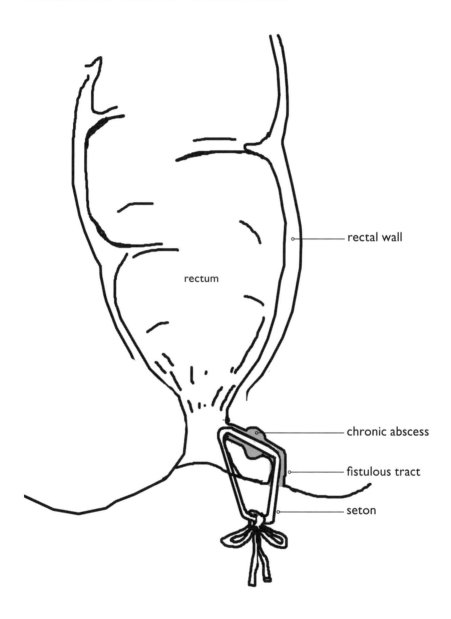

rectal wall

rectum

chronic abscess

fistulous tract

seton

the ends of the fistulous tract don't close before the middle of the tract (where the abscess is likely to be or to have been). A seton is a loop of thick thread or wire that is placed in the fistulous tract to prevent the ends from closing and to allow any pus along the tract to have a place to drain. The seton is placed during a minor surgical procedure and is left in place for as long as needed.

Unfortunately, those people who develop perianal fistulas often get other abscesses and fistulas and need surgery again. Patients with severe perianal disease are often treated by the creation of a colostomy (or an ileostomy if most of the colon is severely diseased and is resected). When this is done, the Crohn's disease in the area that is disconnected usually heals. Unfortunately, if continuity of the bowel is restored, the perianal disease almost always comes back, unless it can be prevented with the use of medication, such as a biological.

Adhesions

Any time a patient has surgery on the GI tract, bands of scar tissue are going to develop afterward. These bands, known as adhesions, will run from the point of surgery to other segments of intestine, to other organs or to the peritoneum (lining of the abdominal cavity), particularly at the site of the previous incision. In most people they do not cause any problems. Adhesions don't hurt. What they can do is fix the intestine at a certain point so that, if it becomes twisted, an obstruction will occur. Most such obstructions get better without surgical treatment. However, some people need surgery to untwist the bowel and cut the adhesions. Of course, new adhesions will form, but usually they will not cause trouble.

Can IBD Come Back After Surgery?
Ulcerative Colitis

If the diagnosis of ulcerative colitis was correct (and it usually is), then a colectomy will be the cure, since this disease occurs only in the colon. If a pelvic-pouch procedure has been performed, then saying the disease is cured is not strictly true, because of the possibility of cuffitis, but that is an uncommon and minor problem. However, unlike Crohn's disease, which has several distinct features, it's important to recognize that doctors have no absolute way to guarantee to someone that they have ulcerative colitis. This means that occasionally a

Bowel Obstruction Caused by Adhesion

Segment of the Small Bowel

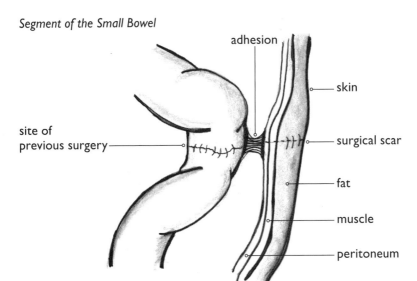

adhesion

skin

site of
previous surgery

surgical scar

fat

muscle

peritoneum

Twisted Segment of the Small Bowel

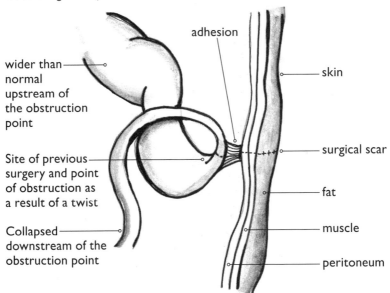

adhesion

wider than
normal
upstream of
the obstruction
point

skin

Site of previous
surgery and point
of obstruction as
a result of a twist

surgical scar

fat

Collapsed
downstream of the
obstruction point

muscle

peritoneum

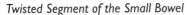

person with ulcerative colitis becomes ill sometime after surgery, and Crohn's disease is diagnosed. Of course, it is possible that that person has had really bad luck, and has had one disease and then the other, but that's considered rare.

Crohn's Disease

Earlier in this chapter, we reviewed the three definitions of "recurrence": endoscopic recurrence, clinical recurrence and surgical recurrence. One of the major areas of research in the past few years has been to try to determine who to treat aggressively to prevent recurrent disease, and who does not need to be treated aggressively.

Some patients are treated with 5-aminosalicylate. The benefits are modest, but the risk of side effects from the medication is extremely low. Many patients who have had more than one resection, or have had a resection but still have residual but inactive disease, are often treated with either azathioprine or 6-mercaptopurine. Recent evidence suggests that anti-TNF drugs may have the best chance of preventing recurrent Crohn's disease.

8

Children with IBD

Both ulcerative colitis and Crohn's disease can begin at any age. However, ulcerative colitis is rare in infancy, whereas Crohn's disease is not unusual. Some 15 to 20 percent of people with ulcerative colitis develop it before the age of 20; in Crohn's disease the figure is 25 to 30 percent.

Research has shown that second-hand smoke increases the risk of Crohn's disease in children, while it reduces the risk of ulcerative colitis. (See Chapter 2 for more on this.)

Diagnosing IBD in Children

Many aspects of ulcerative colitis and Crohn's disease in children are identical to those in adults, but there are some important differences. The symptoms of both diseases seem to be more pronounced in children than in adults. There is also some evidence that children have more intestinal complications (see Chapter 9). However, they have fewer nonintestinal problems than adults.

Most children with ulcerative colitis are diagnosed fairly promptly because blood is found in the stool. The diagnosis of Crohn's disease, however, is often delayed. Improved medical imaging technology has been a major factor in shortening the time it takes to diagnose IBD in children. Doctors and parents have always been reluctant to put children through tests that can be unpleasant, such as multiple blood tests and endoscopy (e.g., colonoscopy, gastroscopy, and so on). Although some blood tests are always necessary, most of the information we need for diagnosis, especially with Crohn's disease, can be obtained with ultrasound and CT scans.

Many children with Crohn's develop the typical crampy abdominal pain, diarrhea and weight loss, but some have only a low-grade fever with few other symptoms. Sometimes it's hard to tell what's going on. Many otherwise normal young children suffer from abdominal pain related to lactose intolerance or constipation, and some children complain about abdominal pain that is a result of emotional stress. Poor appetite and weight loss can lead to an erroneous diagnosis of anorexia nervosa. In some children, the only sign of Crohn's initially is a failure to grow (in medical terminology, this is known as "failure to thrive"); parents and doctors are alerted by the child's small size or delayed puberty. In other children, the initial sign can be an unexplained, persistent fever.

The Issue of Growth

Even after an accurate diagnosis is made, growth failure in children with IBD is a concern. However, we've learned a lot in the past 25 years. We used to think that using steroids to treat the disease was a major factor in delayed growth. The bulk of the evidence now suggests that the major factor is how active the disease is. The more severe the disease, and the longer the time it is active, the more growth will be delayed, even prevented. Steroids *may* play some role in delayed growth, but growth is likely to improve if steroids or other drugs suppress the disease so the child will eat better.

Bone Health

While steroids have become less of a concern in terms of growth, these drugs are still an important risk factor in relation to bone structure and strength, the two main considerations in osteoporosis. Children with Crohn's disease have many interdependent risk factors for unhealthy bones, such as malnutrition, pubertal delay, decreased physical activity and ongoing disease activity. We know that healthy thin people are more at risk for osteoporosis, whereas overweight people are somewhat protected because carrying weight enhances bone strength. Better disease control allows for more food intake (better nutrition) and more physical activity, leading to increased body weight and more muscle mass. Children who are underweight should be encouraged (like all children) to devote part of their leisure time to sports or other forms of physical activity. This is especially important for children with Crohn's disease, as there is evidence that they already have reduced bone formation when they are first diagnosed. This is probably partly due to their genetic makeup but likely also means that the disease was present for many months before diagnosis, and maybe even before the presence of any symptoms or signs of the disease.

Both the frequency and the severity of bone problems are much less in children with ulcerative colitis. When they occur, the risk factors are similar, and so are the solutions.

The diagnosis of osteoporosis in children is more complex than it is in adults. Clinical evidence for both bone fragility (presence of vertebral fractures or repeated fractures of arm or leg bones with minimal trauma, or both) and low bone mineral density must both be present before a child is diagnosed with osteoporosis.

Vitamin D deficiency is well recognized as a standalone, common risk factor for bone disease. Most people in the northern hemisphere have low levels of vitamin D because of limited sun exposure. In addition to this baseline risk, there are three groups of Crohn's patients who are prone to low vitamin D levels due to poor absorption. Children with extensive small bowel Crohn's, or those with extensive resections, or with both, may not have enough surface area for adequate absorption (see page 135, Short Bowel Syndrome). In addition, the few children who have advanced sclerosing cholangitis (see Chapter 9) have reduced absorption due to a lack of bile salts.

Drugs used to treat adult osteoporosis may be used in children; the decision to do so should be made, if possible, by physicians with expertise in this area.

Extra Nutrition for Children with Crohn's Disease

Canadian researchers were leaders in demonstrating that some children with Crohn's disease will grow more if their normal diet is supplemented with nightly feeds of a liquid diet (see Chapter 5). In fact, many children learn to slip small feeding tubes through their noses down into their stomachs each night at bedtime. A bag of an enteral product is hung on a pole and dripped into the tube while the child is asleep. In the morning, the child pulls out the tube and has a normal day. One thousand extra calories or more can be taken in this way. Adults who use liquid-diet therapy for their Crohn's can usually drink the enteral product; children can do the same, but for many it is socially difficult.

Drug Therapy for Children with IBD

Generally, children receive the same drugs as adults, but the doses of some need to be adjusted to body weight, and a few drugs are avoided because they can interfere with the development of certain tissues. Because IBD is often more aggressive in children, many doctors believe that the treatment should also be more aggressive. See Chapter 6 for a discussion of the step-down versus step-up approaches to treatment. In brief, earlier use of the biologicals should be a serious consideration. Steroids are given more frequently to children than to adults, with the knowledge that steroids often work very quickly and lead to improved appetite, weight gain, more energy and resumption of growth, all as a result of rapid disease control. Along with biologicals, the immuno-suppressive drugs azathioprine, 6-mercaptopurine and methotrexate are often considered to be an excellent long-term strategy for children who can't get off steroids, need frequent steroids or need to avoid steroids because of unacceptable or disabling side effects.

One issue that has received a lot of attention in the last few years is that of lymphoma risk with certain IBD treatments. Lymphoma is a collective term for lymph gland cancers. In males in the pediatric and young adult population, a rare form known as hepatosplenic B-cell lymphoma appears to be more likely to occur if azathioprine or 6-mercaptopurine and infliximab (and probably other anti-TNF drugs) are given in combination (see Chapter 6). Before this observation, azathioprine (or 6-mercaptopurine) was frequently the immunosuppressive of choice in this age group. Now, many pediatric gastroenterologists are turning to methotrexate as their first choice or are going straight to anti-TNF therapy. Making the treatment choice even more difficult is a recent study suggesting that early combination therapy with azathioprine and infliximab (and probably other anti-TNF drugs) appears to offer a better response rate than using infliximab alone.

Surgery for Children with IBD

Obviously, the most effective way to reduce inflammation is to remove it surgically. Indeed, doctors tend to be somewhat more aggressive about treating children surgically because of the concern about growth and also because the IBD tends to be more aggressive. Nevertheless, unless puberty has already begun, there is a span of several years in which to suppress the disease and allow growth. No one should jump to the conclusion that children should immediately undergo surgery because their growth is delayed. Not all children with IBD will grow simply because they have surgery; they may just be naturally short. Laparoscopic surgery is particularly attractive, because the scars are much smaller and less noticeable.

In *adults* with Crohn's, 40 percent to 70 percent will need surgery by the 10th year from the time of diagnosis, although these figures are expected to decrease as the benefits of the newer therapies are realized (see Chapter 6). In 2006, a group of American researchers studied close to a thousand pediatric Crohn's patients ranging in age from a newborn to 17 years and found several risk factors that could be used to predict the need for surgery in this age group. The need for surgery was 17 percent at 5 years from the time of diagnosis and 28 percent at 10 years. Some of the risk factors identified were female gender, poor growth at the time of diagnosis and the presence of an abscess, stricture or fistula (these often occur in combination). More recent studies have indicated that a young age at diagnosis combined with small bowel Crohn's disease are additional factors predicting a higher risk of aggressive disease. It is hoped that identification of children at higher risk for needing surgery will facilitate selection of the step-down drug approach for these patients.

When it comes to children with ulcerative colitis, there is much less information about markers of aggressive disease. As in adults, the first attack is often the worst attack. As in adults, some of these patients will not respond to medical therapy and will require urgent surgery. And, as in adults, children who have frequently active disease (which implies poor response to medications) during the first 5 years of disease are likely to require a colectomy.

Psychological Effects of IBD on Children
Children — particularly teenagers — are very anxious not to be seen as different from their peers; their self-consciousness, and the intolerance of other children, often leads to a degree of isolation. Depression and anxiety can occur and may require specific therapies.

Adjustment to an ostomy is particularly difficult; having a "buddy" — another child of similar age who has already adjusted to an ostomy — can help. If a child of similar age isn't available, a young adult is next best. Ask your medical and surgical teams to help you find a buddy for your child.

Most children, like most adults, become tough as a result of having a chronic disease. But this takes time. Parents must try to treat these children the same way they treat their other children. Whenever possible, children with IBD should be allowed to participate in normal activities. Unnecessary dietary restrictions should be avoided. For example, there is no evidence that people with IBD need to avoid junk foods.

It is natural to feel depressed when IBD is diagnosed or when it flares up. Many kids wonder, "Why me?" However, once treatment begins and the symptoms subside, most will perk up. During a flare-up, extra rest may be necessary. When improvement comes, regular activities may have to be resumed gradually.

It is desirable for the child to establish a comfortable relationship with the doctor. Family, close friends and, at times, other patients can be a big help, but the doctor-patient relationship remains extremely important.

Parents and Children, Children and Parents

Most parents can adjust to chronic disease in themselves, and most children can do the same. However, when parents have to adjust to chronic illness in their children, there is sometimes a tendency to be extremely overprotective. At the same time, the sick child goes into denial of the illness and can become resistant to parental intervention.

Parents must try to allow the patient to develop a relationship with the doctor, particularly when the patient is a teenager or a young adult. Parents must give their children a chance to manage their disease independently, in the same way that they must learn to let go as healthy children grow up. By the same token, children should recognize that their parents genuinely care and are trying to help.

Parents, trust your kids. Be there to help them when they want help. Kids, respect your parents. If you want independence, show that you can be responsible. Take your medications without having to be reminded. Tell your doctor (and your parents) when you are sick. Keep your appointments.

9

Complications of IBD

Complications are unforeseen conditions that occur during the course of a disease. Sometimes they arise before the disease is diagnosed and serve as symptoms or signs that lead a physician to the disease. The complications of IBD can be divided into two types: those related to the intestine itself, and those outside the intestine. Here are some of the more common ones.

Complications in the Intestine

Toxic Megacolon

From a medical viewpoint, the most severe complication of any type of colitis is toxic megacolon. The word "toxic" means that the patient is acutely ill with fever, abdominal pain, loss of appetite, diarrhea, nausea and possibly vomiting. "Megacolon" refers to the fact that part or all of the colon is abnormally wide in diameter.

In this condition, the muscular wall of the colon becomes more or less paralyzed. As a result, the gas normally produced by the bacteria in the colon accumulates instead of passing out the rectum. Toxic megacolon is the most feared complication of colitis mainly because it is sometimes associated with perforations in the wall of the colon. The contents of the bowel (including bacteria) can leak into the abdominal cavity, resulting in peritonitis, a condition in which the lining of the abdominal cavity is inflamed. This is a very serious, sometimes fatal, illness. The perforations require emergency surgery. The usual operation is subtotal colectomy, Brooke ileostomy and mucous fistula or closure of the rectum (see Chapter 7).

If there is no evidence of perforation, the standard initial treatment is steroids, often combined with antibiotics, but surgery is frequently necessary. Toxic megacolon can occur with both ulcerative colitis and Crohn's disease of the colon. It is less common in Crohn's colitis because, as the disease progresses, the colon wall becomes thick, scarred and less likely to stretch.

Toxic megacolon is more common in people who have extensive colitis than it is when colitis is limited to a relatively small segment of the colon.

Toxic colitis is similar to toxic megacolon; the main difference is that the colon diameter is still normal. The treatment is usually the same. People having an attack of colitis should not take loperamide, diphenoxylate or codeine to control diarrhea: use of these medications can increase the risk of developing toxic megacolon.

Strictures

Both ulcerative colitis and Crohn's disease can be complicated by strictures, or localized areas of narrowing. Strictures are much more common in Crohn's disease than in ulcerative colitis because Crohn's causes inflammation of the full thickness of the bowel wall. Ulcerative colitis generally involves only the inner lining, so strictures are uncommon.

Strictures may lead to bowel obstruction, which may be temporary (acute) or permanent (chronic). Bowel obstruction is the most common complication of small bowel Crohn's disease. It can occur suddenly or gradually. Sudden or acute obstruction is usually associated with crampy abdominal pain, nausea and, sometimes, vomiting. You may have increased diarrhea, or you may stop passing stool, and even gas, completely. Acute obstruction is not a complication of either ulcerative or Crohn's colitis.

If you have chronic obstruction, which is partial, you will experience abdominal pain, nausea and bloating of the abdomen after meals. The interval between the meal and the symptoms depends on the site of blockage. Less than 1 hour suggests small bowel; more than 1 hour suggests colon. An area of scarring may be dilated (stretched) with an inflatable balloon passed through an endoscope. As noted earlier, improvements in equipment have raised the success rate in experienced hands to as high as 75 percent; relief of obstructive symptoms can last weeks, months or years. If this form of treatment is not possible, or not successful, surgery must be performed.

Perforations, Abscesses and Fistulas

Perforations can occur in both ulcerative colitis and Crohn's disease. Abscesses and fistulas are complications of Crohn's disease only. Just to make it confusing, however, abscesses, and even fistulas, can occur as complications of abdominal surgery for *any* disease.

When perforations develop in the wall of the colon, the bowel contents (including bacteria) leak into the abdominal cavity. If a perforation develops rapidly, the intestinal contents will spill into the peritoneal cavity and cause peritonitis. This is called a free perforation. The vast majority of free perforations in ulcerative colitis occur with toxic megacolon (see page 159). Free perforations can also occur in attacks of severe colitis without megacolon (i.e., toxic colitis), but such events are rare. Free perforations are also rare in Crohn's disease, except with toxic megacolon. The treatment in both ulcerative colitis and Crohn's disease is emergency surgery.

If a perforation develops slowly, the body usually reacts by "walling off" the hole in the bowel wall so that peritonitis does not result. This is called a confined perforation and results in the formation of an abscess (popularly called a boil). An abscess is a walled-off collection of pus. As explained earlier, pus is a mixture of living and dead bacteria and living and dead white blood cells. An abscess can be virtually any size, from tiny and visible only under a microscope to something the size of an orange, or larger.

A fistula, as we've seen, is an abnormal connection between two hollow structures (such as between bowel and bladder, or bowel and vagina) or between a hollow structure and the skin. Once a fistula has been created, by the burrowing nature of the inflammation in Crohn's disease or by drainage (spontaneous or surgical) of an abscess, it is likely to drain intermittently or constantly. Antibiotics are often helpful, but more potent drugs, or even surgery are often necessary.

Perianal Disease

Strictly speaking, this term refers to disease around the anus. But from a practical point of view, it includes disease within the anal canal, as well as around it.

HEMORRHOIDS

Any condition that causes diarrhea or constipation is likely to lead to enlargement of the veins within the anal canal. The enlarged veins are known as hemorrhoids, or piles. They are often felt as soft bumps protruding from the anal canal or immediately around it. Uncomplicated hemorrhoids don't hurt.

Occasionally, a hemorrhoid becomes blocked by a blood clot. This is called a thrombosed hemorrhoid. It causes considerable pain in the region of the anus, and the sufferer will likely be unwilling — or even unable — to sit. The pain is relieved immediately if the hemorrhoid spontaneously ruptures or if a surgeon makes a small cut in it to relieve the tension in the vein wall and surrounding tissues. Either way, there will be a brief but dramatic gush of blood, which always appears to be more than it is. This bleeding is not dangerous and stops by itself.

SKIN TAGS

When hemorrhoids bulge, they stretch the overlying skin. When the hemorrhoids shrink, the stretched skin remains. This is commonly referred to as a skin tag. In Crohn's disease, but not in ulcerative colitis, these tags can become swollen and firm. Once tags thicken, they usually stay that way. They don't hurt, but they can be annoying, especially because bits of stool can get trapped between them, and this can lead to chronic irritation of the skin and itching. However, in most people with Crohn's disease, it is it is believed that surgical removal of these swollen tags can lead to chronic non-healing ulceration of the anal area.

ANAL FISSURES

Many people with hemorrhoids also develop anal fissures. An anal fissure is a cut or tear in the skin of the anal canal. This skin is extremely sensitive, so fissures can be quite painful, especially during a bowel movement and shortly after. The pain is often felt as a stretching or tearing during a bowel movement and as a burning afterward. Most of the pain of anal fissures is due to spasm (excessive contraction) of the anal sphincter, the ring of muscle that opens to let stool out, and stays closed to keep it in. People with Crohn's disease sometimes get fissures that are wider, longer and deeper than those that occur in ulcerative colitis. When a fissure becomes deep, it becomes covered with a layer of pus and may be referred to as an anal ulcer.

ABSCESSES AND FISTULAS
Many people with Crohn's disease develop abscesses and fistulas in and around the anus. You'll find a detailed discussion of how these develop and how they are treated in Chapter 7.

STRICTURES OF THE ANAL CANAL
These are more common in Crohn's disease but sometimes occur with ulcerative colitis as well. If your stools are very loose, you will be unaware of the narrowing. When stools are formed, the diameter of the stool is restricted by the diameter of the stricture. People with strictures have narrow stools, but many people with narrow stools don't have strictures. The simple act of straining to have a bowel movement prevents the anal sphincter from relaxing properly, and this forces the stool to be squeezed out through a narrower passage.

Mild anal strictures need no treatment. More severe strictures may require periodic stretching. This can be done manually with the doctor's gloved finger or with a dilator.

Iron-Deficiency Anemia, Hemorrhage and Massive Hemorrhage
Anemia is a condition in which the blood contains a reduced number of circulating red blood cells. It can be due to a deficiency of iron, folate (a B vitamin), vitamin B12 or some combination of those. But even when these nutrients are present in adequate amounts, some people are anemic simply as a result of having a chronic disease. Chronic inflammation in the body suppresses the blood-producing activity of the bone marrow.

Folate deficiency can occur if you are taking sulfasalazine (see Chapter 6) or if you are severely malnourished. Vitamin B12 deficiency may occur if you have extensive ileal disease, or after surgical removal of the ileum (see Chapter 7). Iron deficiency, however, is a little more complicated.

Anemia due to iron deficiency can develop in one of three ways. You may not be getting enough iron in your diet; this is uncommon but possible, especially if you eat little red meat or organ meats such as liver. Even if you have enough iron in your diet, you may not be absorbing it for some reason. Iron absorption is commonly decreased in people with celiac disease, which is especially common in individuals of Irish descent. If you consume and absorb enough iron but still have iron deficiency, the only other possibility is that you are losing more iron than you are taking in. The way we lose iron is by losing blood. You can lose up to 45 milliliters of blood a day in the stool without seeing anything, if the bleeding comes from high enough up in the GI tract that the blood is thoroughly mixed in with the stool. Losing small amounts of blood on a daily basis can lead to iron-deficiency anemia over a period of several weeks or months.

ANEMIA IN ULCERATIVE COLITIS
No one with a recent onset of ulcerative colitis should have iron-deficiency anemia simply because of the colitis. Even though there is obviously blood in the stool, the amount is almost always less than you think; it takes very little bright red fluid to color a whole bowl of toilet water red. Unless bleeding is truly heavy, the bone marrow is able to use available stores of iron to keep the red blood cell count in the normal range. If you have had several attacks of ulcerative colitis, however, you will likely require iron supplementation, since the stores of iron within the body eventually get used up. Menstruating women are more likely than men to develop iron deficiency, since the menstrual blood loss adds to the loss of iron.

Occasionally, the bleeding is heavier than average and anemia may develop before the body has a chance to respond and produce new red blood cells.

ANEMIA IN CROHN'S DISEASE
Even in the absence of visible bleeding, people with Crohn's disease frequently develop iron-deficiency anemia. There are usually multiple ulcers (open sores) in the small or large intestine, and chronic, continuous, low-grade blood loss is common.

Sudden episodes of visible bleeding can occur, but not often. This happens when an ulcer burrows into a large blood vessel, generally an artery. Fortunately, the normal repair mechanisms of the body usually seal off the bleeding vessel. In some people, sudden bleeding of this type occurs only once; in others, it recurs or becomes persistent, and may require surgical treatment.

If people with extensive disease in the ileum or an extensive ileal resection are not given vitamin B12, they may eventually develop anemia because they may be less able to absorb vitamin B12 (see Common Side Effects of Resection of the End of the Ileum, section on page 132).

MASSIVE HEMORRHAGE

Rarely in Crohn's disease, and very rarely in ulcerative colitis, sudden and massive bleeding occurs. In Crohn's disease, sudden massive bleeding may start in someone who is otherwise feeling well, or during an attack. If the source of such bleeding is the colon, emergency surgery removes the colon, if necessary. If the source of bleeding is the small intestine, the diseased segment will likely have to be removed. Even if bleeding stops spontaneously, the occurrence of a life-threatening hemorrhage usually necessitates removing the diseased bowel to avoid another, possibly fatal, hemorrhage.

Studies have shown that immunosuppressive drugs (such as azathioprine, 6-mercaptopurine and methotrexate) and biologicals (such as the anti-TNF agents) can heal Crohn's disease in some people. If you have had a hemorrhage, your doctor may wish to try to heal your disease instead of advising you to have an operation. The risks and benefits must be carefully considered.

In ulcerative colitis, massive hemorrhage generally happens during a severe attack. Here the inflammatory process goes more deeply into the intestinal wall than usual and disrupts larger blood vessels. Surgical removal of the colon is often necessary.

Complications Outside the Intestine

Inflammatory bowel disease is associated with numerous complications outside the intestines. The areas commonly involved include the joints, the skin, the mouth, the liver, the bile duct, the kidneys, the blood and the eyes.

Painful Joints

Between 10 percent and 20 percent of people with IBD have joint pains at some time. Joint disease associated with intestinal disease is referred to as enteropathic arthropathy. "Arthralgia" means joint pain. "Arthritis" refers to joints that are inflamed (red or swollen, or both). A person with arthritis also has arthralgia, but many people with arthralgia do not have arthritis. I make this distinction because patients with joint pains often say that they have arthritis, yet their doctor does not use this term. But from the patient's point of view, the terminology may not matter much.

Arthritis associated with IBD is nondestructive: that is, the inflamed joints are not permanently damaged, as they are in rheumatoid or gouty arthritis, for example. You may have a lot of pain and swelling, but it is temporary, with no long-lasting effects. One exception to this is ankylosing spondylitis (discussed below).

Typically, arthritis of IBD occurs mainly in the large joints (e.g., knees, ankles) and tends to move from one joint to another. It may flare up when the IBD flares up, and settle down when the IBD settles down. However, it can precede any bowel symptoms by several years and can flare up when the bowel disease is relatively quiet. If the inflamed bowel is surgically removed, this form of arthritis goes away. Of course, if the disease is Crohn's disease and it recurs, the arthritis may recur.

Ankylosing Spondylitis (Sacroiliitis)

This is a type of arthritis involving the sacroiliac joints, with or without involvement of the joints of the spine. You may have pain or stiffness in the lower back, though such symptoms are more often due to ordinary spinal-disc disease. If the disease is looked for with X-rays and other tests, it is found in many people who do not have symptoms. As with arthritis, this condition can precede the onset of bowel symptoms by several years. Unlike arthritis, the symptoms of ankylosing spondylitis (AS), also known as sacroiliitis, do not correlate at all with bowel disease activity and do not improve after surgery on the bowel. Anti-TNF drugs are very beneficial in some cases.

Ankylosing spondylitis can also occur independently of IBD and is indistinguishable from AS in people with IBD. AS occurs in association with Crohn's disease much more than with ulcerative colitis.

BONE DISEASE

Osteonecrosis

The term "osteonecrosis," derived from Greek, literally means "bone death." Osteonecrosis in people with IBD is almost always a complication of steroid therapy. However, it has been reported rarely in IBD patients who have never received steroids. The two most typical locations are the hips and the knees. This condition is extremely uncommon, but it can cause considerable disability. It leads to damage (known as avascular necrosis) of the hip or knee joints and usually requires total hip or knee replacement.

Osteoporosis (Soft Bones)

People with IBD frequently have osteoporosis. Although this is often blamed solely on steroid therapy, it is more likely related to a combination of factors, including low calcium intake, low vitamin D levels, lack of exercise, disease activity and an inherited tendency to develop osteoporosis. Using bone densitometry (also known as BMD, which stands for "bone mineral density"), monitoring of bone health is quite accurate. This test involves a minimal amount of radiation. It is brief (about 20 minutes), painless and safe.

Both calcium and vitamin D are necessary to form bone. As we saw in Chapter 6, vitamin D is available in food and vitamin supplements, and is also produced in the body when the skin is exposed to sunlight. People with Crohn's disease who have had more than 3 feet (about 1 meter) of ileum removed may not be able to absorb enough vitamin D and, possibly, calcium. This makes them susceptible to osteoporosis. The risk increases in postmenopausal women. Measuring blood levels of vitamin D is helpful but, in temperate climates, vitamin D levels can vary considerably with the seasons because of exposure to so much less sunlight during the winter months. There are now several drugs for the treatment of osteoporosis (see Chapter 6).

SORES IN THE MOUTH

About 5 to 10 percent of people with IBD experience intermittent sores in the mouth. These are sometimes indistinguishable from the canker sores (also known as aphthous ulcers) that occur in the general population, but the latter typically occur one at a time, last a few days and then go away. Canker sores in IBD patients often occur in clusters, may be unusually large and may persist for many days, even a few weeks. These sores usually occur when bowel disease is more active.

In addition to ordinary canker sores, people with Crohn's disease

Treating Canker Sores

Here's a treatment proven to be of some value in treating canker sores. You'll need 250-milligram capsules of the antibiotic tetracycline. Dissolve the contents of one capsule in 1 to 2 teaspoons (5 to 10 milliliters) of warm water. Hold the solution in your mouth for 10 to 15 minutes (if you can do it for that long), then spit it out. Try to do this four times a day. Begin this treatment right at the onset of any canker sore, and continue it for a few days. This can shorten the duration of the sore. Apply the local anesthetic viscous lidocaine (available at the pharmacy, without a prescription) directly onto the sores with a cotton swab just before meals to decrease discomfort during eating.

can develop mouth or throat ulcerations that look like Crohn's ulcers in the bowel. Biopsies of these ulcers show microscopic changes typical of Crohn's disease. Steroids may be needed; there isn't a more specific therapy. Fortunately, these ulcers resolve themselves over a week or two in most patients.

A few studies show that people with symptomatic Crohn's disease also have more gum infections and cavities than those whose disease is not causing any symptoms. This may simply be due to a difference in diet; some people with Crohn's disease eat an unusually large amount of refined sugars to replace energy lost by avoidance of other foods.

SKIN DISEASES

Erythema Nodosum

The most common skin abnormality in IBD is erythema nodosum. It occurs in 2 to 10 percent of people with IBD and is somewhat more common in women. It consists of painful, tender red bumps that appear most often on the shins but sometimes show up on other parts of the legs, or even on the arms. It is often associated with an IBD flare-up and usually improves as the bowel disease is treated and improves. Sometimes, erythema nodosum occurs on its own and, at other times, in association with IBD-related arthritis. Although you can try anti-inflammatories such as ibuprofen, most people need a short course of steroids.

Pyoderma Gangrenosum

Pyoderma gangrenosum (PG) occurs in 1 percent to 5 percent of people with IBD and is more common in those with ulcerative colitis. Most people with PG have extensive colitis. PG begins with a raised, red, tender area of skin, which then takes on the appearance of a blister. The roof of the blister breaks down and the result is a skin ulcer. PG usually occurs in multiple locations more or less simultaneously, and the ulcers can be any size, from tiny to extensive. Although these sores are generally painless, they are very unsightly and unpleasant to deal with, and some patients require extensive dressings. Anti-TNF drug therapy may help.

DISEASES OF THE LIVER AND BILIARY TRACT

Fatty Liver

Fatty liver is a common complication in IBD. The cause is unknown, but in most cases it is likely malnutrition. Most patients have no symptoms or signs of the condition, it is not serious and it is usually temporary. However, there are several other causes of fatty liver unrelated to IBD, so tests may be needed.

Primary Sclerosing Cholangitis (PSC)

This is one of the most serious complications of IBD. It occurs in 1 to 4 percent of patients, more often in people with ulcerative colitis than in those with Crohn's disease. Some people with this condition do not have IBD, but about 70 percent do. Primary is a medical term for "unknown cause." Sclerosing means "hardening." This disease causes scarring in the biliary tree (the bile ducts), along with inflammation of the main bile duct or its branches, or of both. The scarring is patchy. It can be present only in the bile duct outside the liver, only in the branches of the biliary tree within the liver or in both locations.

It is well accepted that there are two types of this disease: small-duct PSC and large-duct PSC. The small-duct form is often much less of a problem; it doesn't usually shorten a person's life, and may not cause serious liver damage or progress to large-duct disease and liver transplantation. PSC can be diagnosed by MR; the technique is known as an MRCP (magnetic resonance cholangio-pancreatography). But a more exact evaluation requires an ERCP (endoscopic retrograde cholangio-pancreatography), which involves insertion of a scope down the throat and into the duodenum, and injecting dye into the bile duct. In the small-duct form, these test results will be normal, and a liver biopsy may be done to confirm the diagnosis.

Until the 1980s, no satisfactory treatment, medical or surgical, existed for PSC. Patients died of infection in the liver or of complications of liver damage that eventually results from untreated PSC. In the 1980s, cyclosporine was introduced to the field of transplantation. This drug alone was responsible for moving liver transplants from the back pages of newspapers to the front pages. Because of cyclosporine, the success rate in liver transplants increased from 20 to 80 percent or higher.

Sclerosing Cholangitis

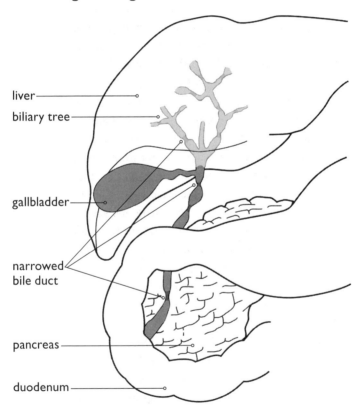

liver
biliary tree
gallbladder
narrowed bile duct
pancreas
duodenum

Thus, since the mid-1980s, the treatment of choice for patients with advanced sclerosing cholangitis has been a liver transplant. Even so, patients with PSC still have a significantly reduced life expectancy compared with IBD patients without PSC, though it is considerably better than it used to be.

The development of new medications for the treatment of other liver and biliary-tract diseases has led to renewed interest in drug therapy for PSC. No drug has yet been proven to arrest or even slow its progression. Studies using a bile acid named ursodeoxycholic acid (ursodiol, or UDCA) have shown that liver blood tests improve, but there is no apparent improvement in the disease itself. Furthermore, a recent study has suggested that ursodiol may increase the risk of bile duct cancer in people with PSC.

Cancer of the Gallbladder or Bile Ducts

Cancer of the gallbladder or bile ducts occurs more often in people with IBD than in the general population. The tumors are more likely with ulcerative colitis than with Crohn's disease. The risk of cancer of the bile ducts is increased in the presence of PSC.

Gallstones

Bile salts are chemicals produced by the liver. They pass down from the liver into the duodenum dissolved in bile and help to digest and absorb fat. Cholesterol is also dissolved in bile. People who have extensive disease in the ileum or have had some of the ileum surgically removed absorb and recycle a smaller percentage of the daily bile-salt output. Since one of the functions of bile salts is to keep the cholesterol in bile dissolved, the reduced level of bile salts allows more cholesterol to come out of solution and form stones in the gallbladder. This applies to those with Crohn's disease only. Currently, no effort is made to prevent these stones from developing. However, many gallstones never cause any symptoms nor require any treatment.

KIDNEY DISEASES

Kidney Stones

Kidney stones, usually composed of either calcium oxalate or uric acid, are much more common in people with IBD than they are in the general population. Most of the increased frequency is in people who have had surgery with removal of bowel.

How Can Kidney Stones Be Prevented?

As with many conditions, prevention is the most desirable route. If someone who has had a resection of some kind has looser stools than normal, increasing oral fluid intake and reducing fluid loss in the stool is a good idea. Ileostomy patients are generally advised to consume at least 2 quarts (about 2 liters) of fluid a day. However, this is not always possible. Using antidiarrheal drugs such as loperamide, diphenoxylate or codeine (see Chapter 6) can be very effective in reducing fluid losses in the stool. Some physicians routinely prescribe low-oxalate diets for patients who have had an extensive ileal resection or those with extensive ileal disease, or both, to reduce the risk of calcium oxalate stones (see Appendix 6).

What If Stones Are Already Present?

Many stones will pass through the urinary tract spontaneously. Stones stuck within a ureter often need to be treated by an urologist, a surgical specialist in diseases of the urinary system. Stones that remain in the kidney are sometimes not treated but monitored with ultrasound. The pain of kidney stones is not always typical. It is usually in the back, but sometimes it is felt in the abdomen, particularly below the waist on one side or the other. This may initially make you and your doctor think that the pain is due to the IBD. If the pain is not like your usual pain, consider the possibility of a kidney stone. If you have stones, a consultation with a nephrologist, a medical specialist in diseases of the urinary system, may be useful. There are treatments that can lead to stones being dissolved, and other treatments that can prevent new stones from forming and existing stones from growing.

Hydronephrosis

The term "hydronephrosis," from Greek, literally means "water kidney." If a ureter is blocked, the pressure on the kidney from the excess urine that cannot pass will cause the urine-collecting system to become stretched. If this persists, the pressure on the kidney can permanently damage it. Most cases occur in people with Crohn's ileitis, due to pressure on the lower end of the right ureter from the inflammatory process. Hydronephrosis is easily diagnosed with ultrasound, and mild cases may improve without surgery.

Amyloidosis

This rare disease causes widespread deposits of an abnormal protein in organs and tissues throughout the body. These deposits damage or destroy cells and interfere with organ function. The abnormal protein is produced by plasma cells, which are one particular kind of white blood cell. Amyloidosis can occur in people who have no other disease, as well as in association with a variety of chronic diseases. When it comes to IBD, amyloidosis occurs mainly with Crohn's disease, and only rarely in people with ulcerative colitis. In most of these people, it will not cause any problems. However, when amyloidosis does cause serious illness, it is generally because it involves the kidneys, with kidney failure as an eventual result. Some experts think that amyloidosis can stabilize or even regress if the IBD is surgically removed, but some studies have shown no benefit at all. For patients in whom the progression of amyloidosis cannot be halted, dialysis and kidney transplantation remain possible alternatives. Other possible treatments are beyond the scope of this book.

EYE PROBLEMS

Eye disease associated with either IBD or its treatment occurs in about 10 percent of patients, though many cases are mild and are not brought to a doctor's attention. There are three main inflammatory conditions: conjunctivitis, episcleritis and uveitis. Cataracts can occur as a complication of steroid therapy (see Chapter 6).

The occurrence of these inflammatory conditions may not correspond to how active the bowel disease is. Inflammation in the eye usually requires local treatment, which is often in the form of steroid drops.

Conjunctivitis (inflammation of the membrane lining, the inner surface of the eyelids and the outer surface of the eye) is the most common condition, but it is not absolutely clear that this is a feature of IBD, since it is also common in the general population. Conjunctivitis can be unpleasant, but it is not serious.

Episcleritis (inflammation of the white of the eye) occurs in 3 to 4 percent of IBD patients, mostly those with Crohn's colitis. Patients usually complain of burning in one eye, and increased tear production. There may be mild localized redness. This condition is also minor.

The uvea is the middle of the three layers making up the wall of the eye. The uvea itself has three components: the iris (the colored part of the eye) at the front, the ciliary body and the choroid. Different people use the term "uveitis" to mean different things. Some people use "iritis" and "uveitis" interchangeably, but iritis is actually one form of uveitis, technically known as anterior uveitis. Iritis occurs in 0.5 to 3.0 percent of IBD patients, mainly in males with ulcerative colitis. It can lead to serious loss of vision and requires treatment by an ophthalmologist. People with iritis suddenly develop blurred vision, headaches and eye pain. In rare cases, this problem can occur repeatedly. There is considerable controversy about how to treat this condition.

BLOOD-CLOTTING ABNORMALITIES

It is well recognized that some IBD patients have abnormalities of the blood-clotting mechanism, resulting in an increased tendency to form blood clots in otherwise healthy blood vessels. There are approximately 13 chemicals known as clotting factors, some of which are increased in certain patients with IBD. In addition, many patients have an elevated platelet count, especially during flare-ups of the bowel disease. Platelets are blood cells that are very important in the formation of blood clots.

Certain conditions predispose many sick people, with a variety of acute and chronic diseases, to develop unwanted blood clots. Patients who are bedridden or dehydrated (whether it be due to fever, vomiting, diarrhea or any other cause) are said to be in a hypercoagulable state, meaning that they are more prone to unwanted clots.

Most of the clots in IBD patients are in veins. The common locations are the leg veins and pelvic veins, but veins anywhere in the body can be involved. To some extent, this problem can be circumvented if you avoid prolonged periods of immobility. People who must stay in bed should be encouraged to wiggle their toes, bend their knees and generally exercise their limbs. Simple strengthening isometric exercises are often very helpful. I always tell my patients that, when visitors come, it should not be just to talk. Visitors should be enlisted to help the patient exercise. Simple things like having the patient push each foot downward against the resistance of another person's hand can be extremely useful. (See Appendix 7 for a set of such exercises.) You can easily make up similar exercises involving the use of other leg muscles or arm muscles. People not confined to bed should be encouraged to get out of bed, even if they don't feel like it.

In some situations doctors give bedridden patients low doses of anticoagulants (blood thinners) to reduce the risk of unwanted blood clotting. The technology for doing this is quite advanced and poses little risk to the patient, even if you are having bloody diarrhea. If you do develop a clot, the usual treatment is an anticoagulant in a larger dose than that used for prevention.

PANCREATITIS

Inflammatory disease of the pancreas has for many years now been reported in association with IBD. Most of the cases are clearly due to certain medications: sulfasalazine, 5-aminosalicylate, azathioprine and 6-mercaptopurine (see Chapter 6). Other cases link pancreatitis with Crohn's disease, independent of any medications, but not ulcerative colitis.

CANCER COMPLICATING IBD

People with either ulcerative colitis or Crohn's colitis have a greater risk of colon cancer than the general population, and people with small bowel Crohn's disease have an increased risk of cancer of the small bowel. Detailed information on this topic is found in Chapter 10.

NUTRITIONAL COMPLICATIONS OF IBD

Malnutrition — characterized by low body weight, sometimes with vitamin or mineral deficiencies — is a common problem with IBD. You'll find details in Chapters 5 and 6 (see also Chapter 7 and Short Bowel Syndrome, below).

Short Bowel Syndrome

People with short bowel syndrome have significant problems with reduced nutrient absorption. They require careful attention to all aspects of nutrition, including water and electrolyte balance. They must be monitored to try to avoid deficiencies. Although a detailed discussion of this condition is beyond the scope of this book, you'll find more details on this condition in Chapter 7.

10

Cancer and IBD

It has been known for many years that people with ulcerative colitis have an increased risk of colon cancer compared with the general population. Some experts think that the cancer risk in Crohn's colitis is probably the same as the cancer risk for ulcerative colitis. People with small bowel Crohn's disease also have an increased risk of small bowel cancer. However, cancer of the small intestine is extremely rare in the general population. Even with the increased risk associated with Crohn's disease, small bowel cancer is still a very uncommon event.

Who Is at Risk?
Ulcerative Colitis
Three factors determine the risk of cancer in people with ulcerative colitis: how much of the colon is (or has been) inflamed, the total duration of the disease and how much of the time the colonic mucosa (inner lining) has been inflamed. The greater the extent of involvement, the greater the duration of disease and the more time that inflammation has been present, the more the risk of developing cancer.

Generally, the more colon involved, the greater the risk. People who have proctitis (colitis limited to the rectum) have a risk equal to that of the general population. Over the past several years we've learned that colon cancer is at least partly genetically determined. There are therefore two groups in the general population: those with no family history of colon polyps (the forerunners of most colon cancers) or colon cancer, and those with a family history of colon polyps or cancer, or both. It is currently believed that a family history of colon polyps or colon cancer, or both, increases the colon cancer risk in people with either kind of colitis.

The risk of cancer is also thought to increase with every year that passes from the time the disease began. During the first 8 years of disease, this risk is just fractionally above that of the general population.

After 8 years the risk rises, but it is still a lot less than we thought it was in the past. Actual numbers aren't given because there is such wide variation in the medical literature.

It has only been in the last 5 to 10 years that researchers have agreed that persistent or frequent episodes of inflammation increase the risk. Inflammation causes increased cell turnover. The more often cells divide, the more chance there is for a genetic "mistake," which can lead to the development of an abnormal cell line. This can be the beginning of a cancer. If this is true, then therapies that *heal* the colon in addition to controlling symptoms should reduce the cancer risk.

Crohn's Disease

The age of the person at the time Crohn's disease first began is felt to be the most important factor in determining cancer risk in people with Crohn's colitis. Those diagnosed before age 20 are at the greatest risk. However, the magnitude of the risk is uncertain. The extent and duration of the disease (independent of age at onset) are likely also factors in colon cancer risk, but these are not as well established as in ulcerative colitis.

As for cancer of the small bowel in people with small bowel Crohn's disease, we still don't know the factors that influence the risk, and the rarity makes it difficult to study.

Reducing Cancer Risk

From the late 1970s, colonoscopy became more and more commonplace and easier and easier to do. It seemed obvious that examining the colon at regular intervals would lead to earlier cancer detection. In the late 1960s, two British pathologists named Morson and Pang described a microscopic change referred to as dysplasia (a change in cell architecture) in the colon biopsies of patients with colitis and early cancer. A progression from low-grade (mild) dysplasia to high-grade (severe)

Biopsy
The word "biopsy" means "to take a tissue sample." It does *not* mean "to look for cancer." If an abnormal area is completely removed, it is an excisional biopsy; if only a piece is taken, it is an incisional biopsy. "Excise" means "cut out completely"; "incise" means to "cut into" something.

dysplasia to cancer was found, and was thought to have some value in predicting which patients were likely to go on to develop colon cancer. Now we know that if the colon is completely removed in people with high-grade dysplasia, about half of them will turn out to have cancer; in some cases it is not visible through an endoscope and can be detected only by a pathologist looking through a microscope. All doctors agree that the finding of high-grade dysplasia means that the colon should be removed. The management of a patient with low-grade dysplasia is more controversial, and beyond the scope of this book.

Just to make matters a bit confusing, sometimes a pathologist will report that a biopsy is "indefinite for dysplasia," which means that the changes are difficult to interpret. Such changes are sometimes due to inflammation, which can make cells look atypical. In fact, inflammation causes cellular changes known as inflammatory atypia. If you have a biopsy that is reported as indefinite, your doctor may want to treat you more aggressively, even if you have few or no symptoms; the goal is to get rid of the inflammation, and then to rebiopsy the area.

Despite these advances, it has been difficult to demonstrate that regular colonoscopies have produced a *marked* reduction in colon cancer occurrence. This has fueled an explosion of new techniques designed to enhance our ability to detect precancer and early cancer. Some of these include spraying dyes onto the mucosal surface during colonoscopy (chromoendoscopy), use of special filters built into the scopes, high-magnification scopes and even confocal laser microscopy, a technique allowing imaging of individual cells with a colonoscope.

Chemoprevention

The term chemoprevention refers to the use of drugs to reduce cancer risk. There is circumstantial evidence that 5-aminosalicylate (5-ASA) (see Chapter 6) can reduce the risk of colon cancer, although the minimum effective dose is unknown. Ursodeoxycholic acid (ursodiol), a drug sometimes given to people with sclerosing cholangitis (see Chapter 9), is also thought to reduce the risk; again, what dose should be used is unknown. Several other medications are believed to have cancer-preventing properties, but all such medications have significant side effects. Cucurmin (a phytochemical found in the spice turmeric) has recently been touted as having preventive properties, but more studies are needed. A potentially undesirable effect of cucurmin is that it can inhibit the effects of anti-TNF medications.

Surveillance Colonoscopy

There are some doctors who feel that surveillance colonoscopy is not worthwhile. But the majority opinion is that it should be done. However, there are varying opinions, even in published guidelines, about when it should be started and how often it should be done.

If most or all of your colon is involved, and the disease has been present for 8 to 10 years, most gastroenterologists will begin surveillance. If currently standard biopsy techniques are used, four biopsies will be taken at 4-inch (10-centimeter) intervals, all the way from the cecum to the rectum. Most people agree that the *minimum* number

---

In the past, doctors' assessment of the amount of colon involved by colitis was based on an X-ray image or a visual abnormality on colonoscopy. However, most people agree that it is more accurate to base the extent of involvement on the microscopic examination of biopsies taken throughout the colon.

Polyps

The word "polyp" simply means "bump." In the general population, there are three main kinds of polyps in the colon. One kind is hyperplastic, and one is neoplastic. The third kind, sessile serrated polyps, are a relatively newly recognized class of polyps. Hyperplastic polyps never turn into cancer, whereas 30 percent of neoplastic polyps (known as adenomas) do turn into cancer (known as adenocarcinoma). Sessile serrated polyps are thought to behave like neoplastic polyps. These types of polyps are no more common, but also no less common, in people with IBD than in the general population. Adenomas typically start to appear after age 40, increasing in frequency with increasing age. If someone has no family history of colon adenomas or colon cancer, they have a 25 percent chance of having an adenoma at age 50. If they do have a family history of an adenoma or colon cancer in one first-degree relative (a parent, sibling or child), they have a 33 percent chance of having an adenoma at age 50. Some people with colitis develop pseudopolyps. The term is misleading because the bumps are real. However, these polyps represent localized areas of inflammation due to the colitis, and the prefix "pseudo" is used to distinguish this type of polyp from the other types.

of biopsies to be taken is 36; some doctors recommend 50 or even more. If any areas look particularly suspicious, your doctor may tattoo the area by injecting a permanent dye, so that the area can be found again, if necessary. The reason for this is that there are very few distinct landmarks in the colon, so it is often impossible to know exactly where you are. If your doctor is using a dye-spray technique, then fewer biopsies may be taken. Patients with total colitis sometimes have significant shortening of their colon; this usually means that the total number of biopsies will be fewer than 36.

Depending on which guidelines you read, surveillance colonoscopy will be done every 2 to 3 years during the first 10 years of disease, every 1 to 2 years during the next 10 years and every year after that. Certain factors are believed to increase cancer risk and result in more frequent examinations. These include sclerosing cholangitis (see Chapter 9) and either frequent or continuously active inflammation of the colon. People with pseudopolyps are also thought to be at extra risk; this may be just because it is harder to identify early neoplastic polyps in the presence of many other irrelevant polyps.

If less than half of the colon is affected by colitis, some gastroenterologists will start surveillance examinations later (typically after 15 years of disease) and may do it less frequently. If the colitis is clearly confined to the rectum and sigmoid, some gastroenterologists don't do surveillance at all; others do. Only when the disease is clearly confined to the rectum is there general agreement that surveillance colonoscopy is not necessary.

What About People with Small Bowel Crohn's Disease?
There is no surveillance procedure equivalent to surveillance colonoscopy for small bowel Crohn's disease. Enteroscopy (endoscopic examination of the small intestine) is impractical and restricted to certain patients. Some gastroenterologists X-ray the small bowel once every few years even if the patient is well, but the chance of picking up an asymptomatic cancer in this way is tiny. Fortunately, small bowel cancer, even in people with Crohn's disease, is very uncommon.

11

Sex, Fertility, Pregnancy and IBD

As with virtually any chronic disease, someone with IBD is concerned about three main aspects of sex: sexual activity, fertility and contraception.

The Effect of IBD on Sexual Activity

Understandably, a disease that has symptoms of abdominal pain, urgent and frequent bowel movements and difficulty getting to the bathroom on time can lead to decreased interest in sexual intercourse for both men and women.

Unfortunately, both doctors and patients tend to avoid talking about sexual activity. However, if a chronic problem is interfering with a sexual relationship, the issue should be considered important enough to warrant discussion and perhaps a change in therapy.

The Impact of Surgery on Sexual Activity

As a result of improved general health after diseased bowel is removed, surgery generally brings an increased libido and improved sexual relationships. However, certain types of surgery clearly produce psychological difficulties.

Most people adapt well to a standard Brooke ileostomy and appliance (discussed in Chapter 7), but concern over body image can result in great anxiety, which in turn can interfere significantly with sexual activity. This is especially true in young singles.

One of the most distressing things that can happen to someone with a Brooke ileostomy is that the appliance can suddenly become dislodged, or can leak during sexual intercourse. Coping with this requires maturity and a "grin and bear it" attitude. Understandably, if this happens even once, the fear that it will happen again is strongly inhibiting. Fortunately, ileostomy appliances have improved significantly over the years, and such events are relatively uncommon. People with a properly functioning Kock (continent) ileostomy are usually not troubled by leaking stool.

Women undergoing total colectomy and ileostomy frequently develop increased vaginal fluid production without signs of infection. In many of these cases, this results in a rather heavy vaginal discharge that is annoying, at least. About one in four women who have had a total colectomy complains of painful sexual intercourse — twice as many as the number of women with this complaint before such surgery. Similarly, men may complain of reduced libido and sexual satisfaction after such surgery. However, despite these problems, the majority of total-colectomy patients report an overall improvement in their sex life.

Men who have a near-total colectomy and pelvic pouch procedure with ileo-anal anastomosis, or a total procto-colectomy to establish a continent ileostomy (Kock pouch), have a 1 to 2 percent risk of impotence. This is because the nerves that control erection are in the same vicinity as those to the anus and rectum; these nerves can be damaged during surgery. There is also a 3 to 4 percent risk of retrograde ejaculation, which means that the semen goes into the bladder instead of coming out of the penis. Because this type of surgery is often associated with mild diarrhea and episodes of incontinence, both men and women who have one of these procedures may feel anxious during sexual intercourse. Nevertheless, as with other types of surgery, sexual life generally improves overall, likely due to better general health.

Fertility

Most studies of patients with unoperated ulcerative colitis have shown no evidence of impaired fertility in either men or women. (For possible fertility problems in women who have had a pelvic-pouch procedure, see Chapter 7.) Not so for Crohn's disease. Women with active Crohn's disease are somewhat less likely to become pregnant, and men with active Crohn's disease who are in ill health or undernourished may have difficulty fathering a child.

We don't know what causes reduced fertility in women with Crohn's disease. It may be that the bowel disease somehow creates blockages of the Fallopian tubes. However, fertility may actually be normal, and the reduced number of pregnancies may be a result of either medical advice to avoid pregnancy or such severe pain with intercourse that it is avoided.

There is some evidence that people with Crohn's disease who are treated surgically may have higher fertility than those who are treated with drugs or diet therapy, or both. Presumably this relates to improved general health. If general health improved sufficiently without surgery, the same improvement might be seen.

Sulfasalazine (see Chapter 6) can reduce the sperm count enough to result in male infertility. Fortunately, this abnormality is reversible, though it takes 2 to 3 months for the sperm count to return to normal after the drug is stopped. None of the other medications commonly used for IBD is known to interfere with fertility. Methotrexate, however, can cause birth defects and miscarriages, so women should stop it at 3 to 6 months before attempting conception.

Contraception
All forms of contraception can be used by patients with IBD. There is no evidence that the birth control pill interacts with any of the medications used to treat IBD, but there is evidence that it *may* aggravate the symptoms of some women with IBD. However, this is controversial and is certainly not a reason to avoid the pill. If you are on the pill and wondering if you should stop it, discuss this with your gastroenterologist.

The Menstrual Cycle and IBD
Recent studies have shown that women with irritable bowel syndrome are likely to experience an increase in their symptoms just before and during menstrual periods. Similarly, many women with IBD complain that their symptoms become worse when they get their period. But this has not been well studied to date, and strategies to help them deal with the problem have not yet been designed.

Pregnancy and IBD

Here are some commonly asked questions, and some answers.

What Effect Can IBD Have on Pregnancy?

Ulcerative colitis and Crohn's disease generally do not have any major adverse effects on pregnancy. Most babies are normal and full term, but about one-quarter of babies born to Crohn's mothers will have a low birth weight. Deliveries are no more complicated than usual and there is no increase in the need for forceps or cesarean section.

If the disease is active before conception, the risks of a miscarriage or premature birth are slightly increased, more so in Crohn's disease than in ulcerative colitis. If a severe attack of IBD occurs during a pregnancy, the chances for a normal delivery and a healthy baby are slightly reduced. If the symptoms of ulcerative colitis first occur during a pregnancy, the chances for a normal delivery and a healthy baby are very good.

Crohn's disease that appears for the first time during pregnancy may have a poorer outcome. However, in comparison with ulcerative colitis, there have been relatively few reports of Crohn's disease beginning during pregnancy. When it has been reported, there has been a significantly higher rate of fetal death.

Does Pregnancy Increase the Risk of a Flare-up of IBD?

For anyone in remission, there is a 30 percent chance of a relapse during the next year. Pregnancy neither increases nor reduces that chance. If a flare-up does occur around this time, it will more likely happen in the first 3 months of pregnancy or soon after delivery. The behavior of the disease during one pregnancy cannot be used to predict what will happen in another pregnancy in the same woman.

Women with Crohn's disease who have had surgery for Crohn's reportedly do much better during pregnancy than those who have never had surgery.

If My IBD Is Active When I Become Pregnant, What Effect Will the Pregnancy Have on the Disease?

If your disease is active at the time of conception, generally it will continue to be active during pregnancy. As when you are not pregnant, therapy should be aimed at controlling the disease.

Can Pregnancy Affect the Course of My IBD?

One study has suggested that women with Crohn's and a previous pregnancy need surgery to remove diseased areas less often than those who have never been pregnant.

What About Abortion and IBD?

There is no evidence that therapeutic abortions carry any greater risks for women who have IBD than for those who don't. If pregnancy occurs while a woman is on the antibiotic metronidazole or on methotrexate, a therapeutic abortion may be recommended. In rare instances, a pregnancy may be terminated in a woman with severe active IBD.

What About Smoking During Pregnancy?

Pregnant women with Crohn's disease who smoke have a higher risk of low birth weight and preterm labor. As it is well known that stopping smoking is beneficial for many people with Crohn's disease, it should be strongly encouraged in this group as well as in all other patients.

Do Women with IBD Need a Special Diet During Pregnancy?

Generally, the typical, well-balanced diet that any pregnant woman should follow is fine. If your disease is active, however, you may have to pay extra attention to your diet. The most important thing is to make sure you are taking in enough energy for the fetus to develop and grow normally. Failure to gain weight at the expected rate is a sign that more energy is needed. Inflammation uses up energy, so extra intake may be necessary. Pregnant patients can be adequately nourished with enteral diets or TPN (see Chapter 5) if necessary.

Can I Take My IBD Drugs When I'm Pregnant?

Like anyone else, IBD patients should try to avoid unnecessary drugs during pregnancy. Fortunately, sulfasalazine has proved safe for the fetus. There is no increased risk of prematurity, stillbirth, fetal deformity or other congenital abnormalities. There is no increased danger of a full-term infant becoming jaundiced if you take sulfasalazine to the end of your pregnancy. But be sure to notify your baby's doctor if you are on sulfasalazine, steroids or narcotic medications.

Published evidence indicates that 5-ASA is relatively safe in pregnancy. There is a slight increase in stillbirths and in preterm delivery, but no increase in fetal malformations. For a long time, steroids were considered safe in pregnancy, but recent studies have suggested that there is a very small risk of fetal deformity over and above the usual risk in the non-IBD population. This doesn't mean you should avoid steroids in pregnancy, only that there should (as always) be a good reason for taking them.

In the past, immunosuppressive medications such as azathioprine and 6-mercaptopurine were generally not recommended during pregnancy, but the current view is that the risk to the fetus, if any, is very small. The thinking is that if you are on azathioprine or 6-mercaptopurine when you become pregnant, and your IBD is under control, you should *not* stop these medications, since disease activity is a greater potential risk to your baby than the drug. As noted earlier, therapeutic abortion may be recommended where the mother has been taking either methotrexate or metronidazole; indeed, methotrexate has been used (in large doses) to produce a therapeutic abortion.

The safety of biologicals in pregnancy, on the fetus, in the newborn and in the growing child is unknown. Based on recent data, some physicians recommend that the monoclonal antibody group (such as infliximab and adalimumab) be avoided after 30 weeks of gestation, but that may not always be practical.

The situation with ciprofloxacin is unclear; it is potentially capable of causing limb and joint abnormalities in the fetus, but there are reports of healthy babies born to mothers who stayed on the drug.

We have limited information about the safety of diphenoxylate and loperamide in pregnancy, and the risk appears to be low. Codeine, the main alternative to these drugs, has been studied more extensively and is associated with a very slight increase in risk to the fetus.

Can I Breast-feed My Baby?
The beneficial effects of breast-feeding are well documented and include a reduced risk of developing IBD later in life. There is no evidence that breast-feeding itself can cause a flare-up of IBD in the mother. If your disease is active at the time of delivery, you may not be able to provide sufficient milk. Sulfasalazine and 5-ASA do make their way into breast milk, but they present no hazard to the full-term infant if you are able to breast-feed. In rare cases the breast-fed infant

Safety of Medications in Pregnancy

Low Risk	Limited Information	Should be Avoided
sulfasalazine 5-aminosalicylate corticosteroids cyclosporine	budesonide azathioprine 6-mercaptopurine ciprofloxacin metronidazole infliximab adalimumab diphenoxylate codeine	methotrexate

Safety of Medications with Breast-feeding

Low Risk	Limited Information	Not Recommended
sulfasalazine 5-aminosalicylate corticosteroids	budesonide infliximab adalimumab	azathioprine 6-mercaptopurine ciprofloxacin metronidazole loperamide diphenoxylate codeine
		Should be Avoided
		methotrexate cyclosporine

has had diarrhea because the mother was taking 5-ASA (tablets, enemas or suppositories).

Steroids and antidiarrheal drugs also make their way into breast milk and may cause side effects in infants. The risk is directly related to the dose. If you want to nurse your baby while you are on any of these drugs, the baby should be carefully monitored by the baby's doctor. Some doctors suggest you should not breast-feed for 4 hours after taking your steroid medication. No information is available on the safety of loperamide during breast-feeding.

It was thought in the past that you should not breast-feed while on immunosuppressive drugs or the antibiotic metronidazole, but there is some evidence that the danger has been overestimated. Nevertheless, these drugs do get into your baby's bloodstream. It may be recommended to reduce your immunosuppressive dosage, and possibly to monitor your child's white blood count. Information about safety of the biologicals is just starting to emerge. Early data suggest that the monoclonal antibody drugs (such as infliximab and adalimumab) do not get into breast milk. These issues should be discussed with your doctor.

12

Self-management of IBD

All patients should consult and discuss with their doctor **before** taking any treatment suggestions outlined in this chapter, or elsewhere in this book, to make sure they are comfortable with the self-management approach and any specific treatment suggestions being considered. The strategies and suggestions listed below are **not** for people who are newly diagnosed. These individuals first need to learn about their condition and get used to how their doctor approaches their particular situation. The treatments suggested here do not ensure success, and it is impossible to canvas every possible diagnosis and treatment scenario. Simply put, medical therapy is not "one size fits all." Finally, it is important to recognize that medicine is a rapidly changing field, and treatment strategies are constantly evolving. **All patients should read the disclaimer at the beginning of this book prior to using any of the treatment suggestions in this chapter or elsewhere in the book.**

The theme of the present is empowerment. In medicine, knowledge is the key to empowerment. The previous chapters provide you with general information about your problem. This one focuses on more personal issues and suggests ways for dealing with these.

Chronic conditions are conditions that can only be controlled, not cured. Common chronic conditions include arthritis, asthma, back pain, diabetes, epilepsy, heart disease, IBD and multiple sclerosis.

Why Self-management?
- You control your life.
- You can travel with confidence.
- You can often avoid delays in treating flare-ups.

Living with these conditions has a significant impact on a person's quality of life and on their careers and family. According to the World Health Organization, chronic conditions will be the leading cause of disability by 2020.

One very useful tool for self-management is what is known as the "patient passport." The Expert Patients Programme, launched in Britain, is another tool, in the form of a training course, that helps patients with long-term conditions take control of their lives. Although the program is not available in North America yet, the five core skills it teaches are available to anyone.

The Patient Passport

The patient passport or patient hand-held record is a passport-sized booklet or card on which a patient records the names and approximate dates of regularly scheduled tests so that they can remind the responsible physician or secretary to schedule tests in a timely fashion. It can also be used to record the dates and results of tests or procedures previously performed. The passport concept was initially created in a number of settings to promote patient ownership and understanding and to improve physician implementation of focused preventive care measures. A personal digital assistant (PDA) can be used in the same way.

Most patients can learn to use a passport, increasing the probability that optimal care will be obtained. Studies have shown that reminders from patients can improve physician compliance for preventive measures. Active patient participation can improve compliance by providing better understanding as to why certain tests are important. An IBD patient passport would provide similar benefits. An example follows (feel free to photocopy the page for your personal use).

Expert Patients Programme

Doctors and patients in Great Britain have been leaders in the study and use of self-management techniques in IBD. In 2001, the government formally recognized the expertise of some laypeople with IBD with the establishment of the Expert Patients Programme (EPP). The

An example of a tailored inflammatory bowel disease passport to facilitate tracking of medications, surveillance colonoscopies, past surgeries, bone mineral densitometry and, possibly, other information. D/C Discontinuation; GI Gastrointestinal.

Ulcerative Colitis / Crohn's Disease Patient Passport

Passport book #:_____

Patient name:_____

Date of diagnosis: _____

Maximum extent of disease: _____

Medications

Drug name	Dosage	Date started	Date and reason for stopping (if applicable)

Bone Mineral Densitometry

Date	Next Appointment

Colonoscopy

Month/Year	Next appointment

Relevant GI Surgery History

Month/Year	Surgical Procedure	Hospital

EPP was launched in 2002 to help patients with long-term conditions take control of their lives. The basis of the program is a training course that teaches people how to manage their conditions by using five core skills:

- problem solving,
- decision making,
- making the best use of resources,
- developing effective partnerships with health-care providers, and
- taking appropriate action.

Before we get into specifics, let's focus on the phrase "developing effective partnerships with health-care providers." *It is important to realize that the idea of self-management is not to abandon your medical team but to help them to help you, by your assuming a certain degree of independence.* For people in remote or underserviced areas, your team may be just you and your family doctor. At the other end of the spectrum are people who get their care at centers for IBD; in that setting, there are often multiple team members, including a group of gastroenterologists, a nurse-practitioner and a research coordinator. This team may also include one or more surgeons, and a variety of specialists, depending on the patient's needs — for example, a rheumatologist (arthritis specialist), a dermatologist (a skin specialist), a nephrologist (a kidney specialist) and others. In some places, the administrative assistants of these various doctors are also knowledgeable, often have the task of triaging a problem, and may sometimes give advice. Even if you have such a team supporting you, not to be forgotten is your family doctor, who should be receiving reports from all these people. Having IBD doesn't make you immune to any other medical problems, and your family doctor will often be on the front line for assessing, diagnosing and treating such problems, or arranging an appropriate referral.

If you want your doctors to help you, you have to help them to help you. For example, you may not take one or more of your medications for various reasons — you're feeling better and think you don't need the medication; you just plain forget; you take so many medications that you're angry and frustrated and decide not to take the one you hate the most; you run out of pills and don't bother to get them renewed. Clearly, none of these is in your best interest; as I've said, you are an important member of your treatment team.

Practical Information: Tricks of the Trade
Ulcerative Colitis
Ulcerative colitis attacks vary in their intensity; they may be mild, moderate or severe. Below I define and outline some treatment options for such attacks; first, though, it's important to understand what certain terms mean. When a person has colitis, they have to make frequent, urgent, unpredictable trips to sit on the toilet. When they get there, nothing may come out, or there may be a little "wet gas" or a little blood and liquid stool, or more of a bowel movement. For our purposes, the number of "trips to the toilet" means each time you go to sit on the toilet, regardless of what comes out, even if it's nothing. When nothing comes out, we refer to that as a "false urge." If you sit on the toilet and stay there for half an hour, it's just one trip. The number of times a person goes to sit on the toilet is a more useful concept than the number of bowel movements, if you think of a bowel movement as the passage of stool. Some people with colitis will not have any sizable bowel movements.

MILD ATTACK
Definition:
- two to five trips to the toilet in 24 hours,
- small amounts of blood,
- mild urgency,
- little or no need to get up from sleep to sit on the toilet,
- good appetite,
- no fever, and
- normal energy.

Treatment Considerations:
- sulfasalazine or 5-ASA — start or increase oral dose; and/or
- rectal therapy:
  - 5-ASA suppositories or enemas;
  - hydrocortisone foam/liquid enemas or budesonide liquid enemas;

If you are having an attack of colitis, do not take medications such as loperamide, diphenoxylate or codeine to control diarrhea. Use of these medications can increase the risk of developing toxic megacolon (see Chapter 9).

- combination of above;
- other treatments as agreed upon with your doctor.

MODERATE ATTACK

Definition:
- 5 to 10 trips to the toilet in 24 hours,
- moderate amounts of blood,
- moderate urgency,
- up from sleep one to two times some nights to sit on the toilet,
- reduced appetite,
- with or without fever,
- reduced energy.

Treatment Considerations:
- It is best to call your doctor.
- If you are on a biological (e.g., anti-TNF), you may be eligible for an "early" dose.
- You may be a candidate for a clinical trial.

If you are on antibiotics or were within the past 3 months, or have recently traveled to the tropics or a developing country, tell your doctor.

If (and only if) you are an experienced patient, and you have previously cleared this kind of self-management with your doctor:
- Consider increasing your dose of oral 5-ASA.
- Take acetaminophen for fever over 100°F (37.7°C).
- Monitor your symptoms carefully, and *get in touch with your doctor ASAP.*

If you *must* start therapy on your own, oral steroids is the usual choice — prednisone, or prednisolone, 40 milligrams daily. If already on steroids, double your dose or go to 60 milligrams daily, whichever is less. *Get in touch with your doctor ASAP.*

SEVERE ATTACK

Definition:
- 10 to 20+ trips to toilet in 24 hours,
- heavy blood,
- moderate to marked urgency,
- up from sleep every night to sit on the toilet,
- reduced appetite,
- with or without fever,

- reduced energy.

Treatment Considerations:
- Call your doctor immediately.
- If you can't speak to your doctor, go to the hospital.
- If you are on a biological (e.g., anti-TNF), you may be eligible for an "early" dose.
- If you are traveling, go to the largest nearby hospital, preferably a university-affiliated hospital (see the IAMAT listing in the Resources section on page 236, or contact the local Crohn's and colitis chapter)

If you are on antibiotics or were within the past 3 months, or have recently traveled to the tropics or a developing country, tell your doctor.

Crohn's Disease

Self-management of Crohn's disease is a little more complicated than that of an attack of ulcerative colitis. Some flares of small bowel disease simply cause obstruction (blockage); others cause crampy abdominal pain and diarrhea. Even in a person who has Crohn's in both the small bowel and the colon, the disease can flare up in one location and not the other.

OBSTRUCTIVE FLARE — MILD
Definition:
- feeling "off," nausea, decreased appetite;
- crampy abdominal pain;

Are You Dehydrated?

Here's a simple way to judge if you're dehydrated. If you have to urinate only once or twice a day, and the volume of urine passed is small and the urine is yellow or darker, you are likely dehydrated. If your urine is a rich yellow, you are probably mildly dehydrated; if your urine is the color of weak tea, you are moderately dehydrated and should go to a hospital, where you probably will receive intravenous fluids; if your urine is the color of strong tea or cola, you are severely dehydrated and *must* go to a hospital and receive intravenous fluids. If you urinate four or five times a day, and urine volumes each time are large, and the urine is colorless or the color of straw, dehydration is unlikely.

A minimum normal urine output is 16 ounces (500 milliliters) every 24 hours. A desirable urine output is 32 to 48 ounces (1,000 to 1,500 milliliters) daily.

- may be a burst of diarrhea, then no bowel movements or gas.

Treatment Considerations:
- Have nothing to eat or drink for 3 to 6 hours;
- Then take clear fluids for 36 hours, then progress diet;
- Monitor your urine output — if you think you're dehydrated, you need to increase your fluid intake; if you can't, go to the hospital.

OBSTRUCTIVE FLARE —MODERATE

Definition:
- feeling "off," nausea, markedly decreased appetite;
- severe crampy abdominal pain,
- may be a burst of diarrhea, then no bowel movements or gas.

Treatment Considerations:
- Call your doctor or go to the hospital.

If (and only if) you are an experienced patient and you have previously cleared this kind of self-management with your doctor:

1. Have nothing to eat or drink for 3 to 6 hours.
2. Then take clear fluids for 36 hours, then progress diet or enteral diet (see page 199);
3. Monitor your urine output — if you think you're dehydrated, you need to increase your fluid intake; if you can't, go to the hospital.

- For pain management: you may take acetaminophen with codeine at the beginning; no narcotics after that unless directed by your doctor.
- If not improving or getting worse, *call your doctor or go to the hospital.*
- If you *must* start drug therapy on your own, start steroids (prednisone, prednisolone or budesonide) *or* double steroids, up to a

---

What to Do If a Flare Is Atypical

If —
- your flare-up is different than usual,
- your flare-up is worse than usual,
- your pain worsens after first 6 hours,
- your pain becomes steady,
- you weren't vomiting, and you start vomiting,

Go to a hospital.

maximum of 60 milligrams of prednisone or prednisolone daily. Doubling budesonide is not useful; your doctor may temporarily switch you to prednisone or prednisolone. *Get in touch with your doctor ASAP.*

OBSTRUCTIVE FLARE — SEVERE

Definition:
- feeling very unwell;
- loss of appetite;
- severe abdominal cramps;
- may be a burst of diarrhea, then no bowel movements, or gas;
- nausea and vomiting.

Treatment Considerations:
- Call your doctor immediately.
- If you can't speak to your doctor, go to the hospital.
- If you are on a biological (e.g., anti-TNF), you may be eligible for an "early" dose.
- If you are traveling, go to the largest nearby hospital, preferably a university-affiliated hospital (see the IAMAT listing in the Resources section on page 236, or contact the local Crohn's and colitis chapter)

NON-OBSTRUCTIVE FLARE — MILD

Definition:
- mild abdominal cramps,
- diarrhea,
- no fever (temperature under 99.1°F/37.3°C),
- little or no need to get up from sleep to sit on the toilet,
- good appetite,
- normal energy.

When's the Best Time to Check Your Weight?

Everyone's weight fluctuates during the day, and tends to be highest in the evening and lowest in the morning. The most accurate time to weigh yourself is first thing in the morning, after you urinate, before you get dressed, and before you eat or drink anything. It is not useful to measure your weight more than once a day.

Treatment Considerations:
- Take clear fluids for 36 hours, then progress diet.
- You *may* start or double 5-ASA, and maintain for 2 to 4 weeks, then taper back to usual dose.

If (and only if) you are an experienced patient and you have previously cleared this kind of self-management with your doctor:
- You may start budesonide; if on it, and less than 9 milligrams daily, it can be increased to 9 milligrams.
- Following an enteral diet (see page 199) instead of steroids is a choice for some.
- If on prednisone or prednisolone, double your dose for a few days (to a maximum of 60 milligrams), then return to your usual dose, with a quick taper or without a taper.
- You may be a candidate for a clinical trial — call your doctor.
- Monitor your symptoms carefully, and *get in touch with your doctor ASAP.*

NON-OBSTRUCTIVE FLARE — MODERATE OR SEVERE
Definition:
- moderate or severe abdominal cramps,
- diarrhea,
- fever,
- need to get up from sleep to sit on the toilet
- reduced appetite,
- reduced energy.

Treatment Considerations:
- Call your doctor or go to the hospital.
- If you can't speak to your doctor, go to the hospital.
- If you are on a biological (e.g., anti-TNF), you may be eligible for an "early" dose.
- If you are traveling, go to the largest nearby hospital, preferably a university-affiliated hospital (see the IAMAT listing in the Resources section on pages 237–238, or contact the local Crohn's and colitis chapter)

If you are on antibiotics or were within the past 3 months, or have recently traveled to the tropics or a developing country, tell your doctor.

How to Use an Enteral Diet

You are having an ongoing flare-up of your Crohn's disease, but you are not sick enough to be in the hospital. You have decided you don't want to take steroids this time but that you would like to try a nutritionally complete liquid diet instead.

The cost of liquid diet products is a concern to some people. Keep in mind that you will not be eating "real food," so you'll be saving money on that. Furthermore, some governments and drug plans will pay the cost of the liquid diet if your doctor verifies that is your sole source of nutrition.

If (and only if) you and your doctor have agreed that you can use liquid diet therapy, there are a few things you need to do or know to make it nutritionally adequate and reasonably safe. First, you must use what is known as a nutritionally complete diet. Your doctor can tell you which products are nutritionally complete. Liquid diets, when taken properly, supply all the carbohydrate, protein, fat, vitamins and minerals your body needs. However, there is one thing that these diets do not supply adequately, and that is water. If you are going to live on an enteral diet, you must supplement it with clear fluids. Take a clear fluid when you are thirsty, and take a clear fluid when you have taste fatigue (bored with the taste of the enteral diet). By doing this, you will allow your body to maintain its normal chemistry.

Second, you need to know your target weight, so that you can calculate your caloric goal. If you are near or at your normal weight, use that. If you have lost more than 10 pounds (about 5 kilograms), you should not use your original weight for your calculations because it is unlikely you will be able to consume the amount of the liquid diet needed to reach that goal. On the other hand, you should not use your current weight because you will then probably only maintain that weight and not gain back the weight you have lost. What I usually advise is to choose a weight halfway between your current weight and your original (normal) weight. Discuss your target weight with your doctor.

Third, you need to know how to calculate your nutritional needs. The tables on page 200 give you the basic information. They are just guides; talk to your doctor about your specific requirements.

Fourth, you need to know what product you are going to use and its caloric value per container. Taste testing has shown that more people prefer the "plus" products. Most of these products contain 360 calories per 8 ounce (250 milliliter) container.

A Guide to Nutritional Support (1)

A healthy person doing . . .	Needs this number of calories per pound body weight
light activity (desk job)	10
moderate activity (on your feet)	15
heavy activity (construction)	20
Sick outpatient	add 2–3 calories
Sick inpatient	add 4–5 calories

A Guide to Nutritional Support (2)

Calculate your needs *Assume that you will get 300 calories a day from clear fluids*
Aim for 25% of your caloric goal on Day 1
Aim for 50% of your caloric goal on Day 2
Aim for 75% of your caloric goal on Day 3
Aim for 100% of your caloric goal on Day 4

And finally, you need to know how to drink these products. If you drink them at the same speed that you would drink a glass of juice, you will probably feel bloated and nauseated, and you may get more diarrhea. At least for the first few days, you need to sip these products *slo-o-o-wly*. How slowly? Take 30 to 60 minutes for 8 ounces (250 milliliters). After the first few days, some people will be able to drink these products at a more normal speed. However, there is no rush.

Case Example

Let's say your normal weight was 150 pounds and you currently weigh 130 pounds. Let's also say that you are a moderately busy person, spending a lot of time on your feet. Multiply 140 pounds (your target weight, halfway between 130 and 150 pounds) by 15 calories per pound (see table 1), for a total of 2,100 calories. You are not sick enough to be in the hospital, so let's add 2 calories per pound (140 multiplied by 2), which equals 280 calories. Your total caloric requirement per day is therefore 2,100 plus 280, for a total of 2,380 calories. Assume 300 calories a day from clear fluids, leaving you with a caloric goal from the enteral diet of 2,080 calories a day. If you are using a plus product providing 360 calories per container, you will need to drink about six containers a day. Many people initially say, "*Six* containers a day! How can I possibly do that?" You'll find, though, that if you are not eating solid food, it is really not that difficult. Assuming that you sleep 8 hours a day, you'll have 16 hours to drink six containers plus clear fluids.

See Chapter 5 for more information on liquid diets.

If You Have an Ileostomy or Short Bowel Syndrome, or Both

If you have an ileostomy, short bowel syndrome, or both, you need to pay attention to your fluid intake and urine output. If your small intestine has *not* been shortened by surgery, you should expect your ileostomy output to be less than 1 liter a day. Because the length of a "short bowel" is different for different people, it's not possible to specify how much stool output is acceptable. A desirable urine output is at least 48 ounces (1.5 liters) a day. Less than 16 ounces (500 milliliters) a day is abnormal. Many people with ileostomies or short bowel are chronically dehydrated; the result of this is that they have a markedly increased risk of kidney stones compared with the general population. These stones can develop and grow without causing any symptoms, until, one day, you have a problem. It is a good idea to measure your 24-hour urine output on a few occasions, so that you know whether your output is adequate and also become familiar with what is desirable so that you don't have to keep measuring the volume.

Taking Care of Your Bones

Many adults develop osteoporosis as they get older. As mentioned earlier, the use of steroids such as prednisone to treat IBD increases the risk, and although calcium can be added to the skeleton easily up to the age of 35, after that age it becomes more difficult. Ingesting enough calcium to prevent further deterioration seems to be effective, but medications may also be needed to treat, or try to prevent, osteoporosis (see Chapter 6). See Appendix 3 as a guide to desirable calcium intake.

Following a Low-Lactose or Lactose-Free Diet
If you want to avoid lactose to see if that reduces your cramps and diarrhea, consider trying a low-lactose diet. (See the discussion on this topic in Chapter 5.) If your diet contains few milk products to start with, or if avoidance of milk and milk products produces only a partial benefit, it may be worthwhile trying a lactose-free diet, to see whether further benefit can be achieved (see Appendix 2).

Maintaining Nutrition
Whether or not you are having a flare-up, it's important to make sure you're meeting your daily nutrient requirements. You'll find plenty of information and tips on how to do this in Chapter 5 and also in Chapter 6 (in particular, the sections on vitamins and minerals), as well as the information provided below.

If You Need to Gain Weight
The first thing you need to know if you need to gain weight is where the calories are. The table below is a simple guide.

Food Source	Caloric Density (calories per gram)
Carbohydrates (e.g., bread, pasta, potato)	4
Protein (e.g., meat, fish, eggs)	4
Fat (e.g., animal fat, vegetable oils)	9
Alcohol	7

When you're trying to gain weight, it is generally harmless to eat an increased amount of fat. I am not suggesting you eat a high-fat diet all the time, since fat may increase the risk of heart disease and other diseases in some people. But when I have a patient who is having trouble gaining weight after a flare-up of IBD, I often suggest high-fat, high-energy foods such as bacon and eggs, potato chips, various fried foods, cake and ice cream. Remember, it is extremely difficult to gain weight if you avoid fat. You have to eat more than twice as many grams of carbohydrate and/or protein for every gram of fat that you avoid. Most people who eat a very-low-fat diet will lose weight, no matter how much they eat.

What to Do If You Suffer from Fecal Incontinence

Fecal incontinence — having a bowel movement before you get to a toilet— is an embarrassing and frustrating problem for people who have it. Antidiarrheal drugs (see Chapter 6) will help, as long as you are not in the middle of a flare-up of your disease. Also check with your local Crohn's and colitis association to see if it distributes "can't wait" cards. Many restaurants and other establishments recognize these cards and allow people to the establishment's bathroom even if they are not going to be using its services.

What to Do When You Are in the Hospital

Hospital Food

Hospital food is often the source of jokes, sometimes on quality, sometimes quantity, and often both. "This is *not* what I asked for!" is a common refrain. Part of the problem is that many hospitals contract out their food service. You fill out a menu card, and a nutrition technician collects the card. Your card may or may not be reviewed by the hospital dietitian. The food requests go to an outside facility, and a large food order is then sent to the hospital for distribution. It is clear that part of the problem is that with so many steps, orders are bound to be mixed up.

When you are fighting an illness, your body needs energy for that fight. There is no magic biological source for that energy — it comes from the calories in the food you are eating. If you don't provide your body with enough energy, your body will use your own tissues (mainly your muscles and fat) to get that energy.

How to Get Adequate Nutrition

Many hospital tests require you to fast for several hours; others require that you be on a clear fluid diet. Often, a test will have to be delayed, for a variety of reasons. It's important for both you and your doctor to remember that you should not be on clear fluids for more than a few days, unless there's no choice. If you are being kept on a restricted diet, ask your doctor to order a vitamin pill.

You can't afford to be fussy. "I don't like the food" is not acceptable, unless family or friends are bringing you food. If your diet is restricted for medical reasons, make sure that your doctor approves of food being brought in, and also that whoever is bringing the food is aware of the restrictions.

You may not be able to eat everything on your tray at mealtime. If at all possible, remove anything that you might eat or drink later, and send the tray back as empty as possible. Use the leftovers for between-meal snacks.

How to Eat in the Hospital

Many people who eat or drink while lying in bed become nauseated. If you are nauseated, tell your doctor. There are many causes for nausea, especially in hospitalized patients. However, if the nausea is from being in bed all the time, you may be able to solve the problem. Whenever you drink anything, sit up, with your legs dangling off the bed (or sit in a chair), and try to stay upright for at least 30 minutes. Whenever you eat anything, sit up, with your legs dangling off the bed (or sit in a chair), and try to stay upright (sitting, standing or walking) for at least 60 minutes. If the nausea persists, your doctor may prescribe medications to reduce acid or to assist stomach emptying, or both.

Activity in the Hospital

When you are in the hospital, try not to think of it as a prison. Get permission to go outside, weather permitting. Having an IV line, including a central line, does not mean you have to stay indoors. Even patients with various drainage tubes, drainage bags, bladder catheters and other devices can go out. If you are on a tube feeding, don't be embarrassed and hide in your room. Getting out into fresh air (and even polluted air!) improves outlook. Whether it's roaming the halls of the hospital or strolling outside, remind yourself that exercise is good for you. The more you strengthen your muscles, the more rapidly you will recover from the illness or operation that has led to your hospitalization. I give my hospitalized patients and their families a set of isometric exercises to help them regain or maintain strength (see Appendix 7).

If you are weak, the philosophy should be that any activity is better than no activity. Lying in bed, even if the head of the bed is raised, uses no muscles whatsoever. Sick people become very weak very fast. I tell patients who are very weak to start by just sitting on the edge of the bed with their legs dangling. The next step is to stand beside the bed, then sit, then stand again. After you have mastered that, the next step is to get out on one side of the bed, walk around the bed and get in on the other side. Walk to the doorway of your room and back. Don't be embarrassed about doing little bits of exercise at a time. It is much better for you to do lots of little bits of exercise many times a day than to take one huge walk once a day and then have to spend the rest of the day lying in bed, doing nothing, and recovering from overdoing it. I have had patients start out with limited activity such as this and end up literally running up and down the stairs of the hospital — carrying an IV pole! *The bottom line for your muscles: Use them or lose them.*

Being active has psychological rewards as well as physical ones. And there are other things you can do for yourself in the hospital to make it feel more like home. Have family or friends bring your schoolwork, office work or other work, and your laptop or other portable computer devices (insured). Wear your own clothes, use your own pillow and have someone bring you soft toilet paper. Get your visitors to help you do your exercise. You are not in the hospital to entertain them.

13

Living with IBD

In the preceding chapters, we've covered various issues specific to IBD. This chapter provides an overview of the kinds of problems and concerns faced by many people with chronic illnesses, as well as coping strategies and other tips to improve one's quality of life.

Life Expectancy

Over the past 40 years, the life expectancy of people with IBD has approached that of the general population. This is attributable to several factors, including earlier diagnosis, a greater range of therapies, better attention to nutrition, better surgical techniques and much better care following surgery.

From a statistical point of view, the first attack of either type of colitis is often the worst the person will experience. The risk of dying from any attack of acute colitis has become extremely low. In fact, the only measurable risk is associated with first attacks.

Ulcerative Colitis: What Happens?

Of people who initially have ulcerative proctitis (inflammation in the rectum only), between 10 and 20 percent can expect to progress to more involvement of the colon, usually within the first 2 years but occasionally even after that. Of those who have ulcerative colitis involving the rectum and sigmoid colon, up to 50 percent may progress to more involvement of the colon, usually during the first 10 years of disease. The percentage of people dying from ulcerative colitis has steadily declined over the past 40 years; the risk is greater than that of the general population only with the first attack. The lifetime risk of requiring colectomy is about 30 percent. However, more people with extensive colitis will need surgery than those with limited disease. It's impossible to predict a person's disease pattern. You can have frequent flares in one year, then no flares for 10 or 20 years, or even longer.

Crohn's Disease: What Happens?

Studies over the years have consistently shown a higher mortality risk in Crohn's disease than in ulcerative colitis. However, just as the risk of dying from ulcerative colitis has decreased greatly in the past 40 years, the same is true for Crohn's disease. It is currently thought that the mortality risk is close to that of the general population. There appears to be a modest increase in this risk in three patient groups: those people who are in the first 5 years of the disease, people who require multiple operations and those whose disease begins at a young age.

In the long term, patients with Crohn's disease can expect surgery much more often than those with ulcerative colitis. Among people with all forms of Crohn's disease, the probability of requiring some kind of surgery is about 70 percent. The average number of operations per patient in this group is approximately three. But these statistics include minor operations, such as draining a perianal abscess. It appears that the recent introduction of the medications known as biologicals significantly reduced these numbers.

Although the average person with Crohn's can expect to be sick more often than someone with ulcerative colitis, the pattern of the disease in many individuals is impossible to predict, just as is the case for ulcerative colitis.

Patients with small bowel Crohn's disease who have had more than 3 feet (about 1 meter) of ileum removed are much more likely to have gallbladder stones or kidney stones, or both, than the general population, or than patients with Crohn's disease who have not had this extent of surgery.

Quality of Life with IBD

Quality of life has become an important measuring stick for evaluating the effects of chronic diseases, and of various treatments. In the 1980s, a group at McMaster University in Canada developed a quality-of-life index to evaluate patients with IBD. This index has been used in a variety of studies, all over the world.

However, while statistics can be very helpful, in the end it comes down to each individual. A drug or surgical procedure that benefits most patients may not be looked on favorably by a given person. Furthermore, in studying any treatment choice, measuring the quality-of-life index over a period of time is desirable.

Case Example

Let's take someone who has been continuously ill with Crohn's disease for several months. She is chronically fatigued, eating poorly and taking multiple medications. Surgery is advised and performed. One month after surgery, she is feeling much better, is off almost all medications and is eating well, and her quality of life is clearly much improved. She does have diarrhea, which is a result of the surgery, but she has been told that this is usually temporary and so she is optimistic.

Six months later, the diarrhea has not gotten any better, and she is now being told that this diarrhea — a result of surgery, not of Crohn's disease — is likely to be permanent, and that medication will be necessary to keep it under control. A quality-of-life measurement taken at this point is not as good. Three months later, she develops symptoms indicating that the Crohn's disease has recurred. Over the next few weeks she does poorly, develops an abscess and is told that another operation will be necessary. At this point, her quality of life is greatly colored by what has happened and what is going to happen, and the score is significantly reduced.

After the second operation, the patient is pessimistic. But as it turns out, there is no evidence of recurring Crohn's disease for the next 5 years. As the woman acclimatizes to chronic diarrhea requiring antidiarrheal therapy, her quality-of-life score steadily improves.

Factors Affecting Quality of Life

LOSSES

Developing a chronic disease may mean certain losses for the sufferer. If the disease is mild, losses will be minimal. However, if you are frequently or continuously ill, the effects on life in general are likely to be significant. Unfortunately, personal relationships frequently suffer. It is not unusual for a healthy spouse to be unable to cope with chronic illness in a partner. Unmarried patients generally find it more difficult to establish lasting relationships. They may be embarrassed about the disease, or unable to participate in various activities because of restrictions the disease places on them. Or, they may lack sufficient energy to engage in certain activities with a potential partner.

Having a chronic illness sometimes means a loss of independence. If you are frequently ill, and especially if your illness requires hospitalization, you may need to depend on someone else to deal with simple chores. One of the hardest things for most patients is loss of the ability to control their own lives, even if temporary.

ANGER

When older people develop a chronic illness, they may be upset, but they tend to accept it more easily than young people. As people get older, they see family and friends developing illnesses and expect to have some sort of problem sooner or later. Conversely, young people generally assume that everyone else in their age group is healthy, and their feeling is "Why me?" Of course, it's not true that all young people are well. Many young people have friends who have severe asthma and end up in emergency departments on a regular basis. Others have friends with severe diabetes who must inject insulin every day. Still others have friends who have leukemia or some other form of cancer. Nevertheless, it is true that most young people are healthy, and certainly the image of youth is constantly linked with the idea of health and energy in our culture. So, it's okay to be angry.

Particularly in the initial stages of disease, you are likely to feel anger toward family, friends and health-care workers, all of whom are trying to be helpful but cannot know exactly how you feel. Even when they are coping well, some patients are angry and frequently feel that people —be it parents, teachers, coworkers, relatives and friends — don't understand what they're going through. To some extent, this perception of a lack of understanding is accurate. Even if teachers or coworkers are told the name of the disease (and patients don't always want to advertise their problems), many have no good understanding of what effects such diseases have on a person's life.

Especially when IBD is resistant to treatment, you may feel that days are like weeks and weeks are like months or years. You may temporarily lose confidence in your ability to overcome an attack of the illness. Beware. This pessimistic attitude and frustration with the disease may lead you to ignore treatment instructions, or at least to be careless about them. This is understandable but clearly not in your best interest.

Coping Strategies

If you have a chronic illness such as Crohn's disease or ulcerative colitis, there are many ways you can improve your situation and develop a more positive outlook.

First, accept the fact that you have the disease. Then learn about it. Learn about the treatments. Think of yourself and your health-care providers as a team. Help them to help you; in this way you will help yourself. As is often said, no matter the problem, take one day at a time.

When you feel well, eat well. Consider that a little extra weight is like money in the bank. Unless you are clearly overweight, don't worry about gaining a few extra pounds. When your disease flares up and you lose weight, you will not be as badly off.

If you know that antidiarrheal drugs effectively control your diarrhea or the urgency to go the bathroom, use them to give you psychological security when you are going out, whether to the theater, a sports event, a party or simply the grocery store. Similarly, such medications can be helpful in sexual activity.

Be self-reliant. Learn which kinds of medical decisions you can make on your own. Don't feel that you have to ask your doctor everything. This will build your self-confidence and help to make you feel better. See Chapter 12 for more information on this topic.

Financial Effects of Chronic Disease

Perhaps one of the most difficult areas in maintaining quality of life is the financial burden of chronic disease. Health plans may take care of hospital costs and a few outpatient expenses, but some people don't have a health plan, and others have plans that cover only part of the cost of medications, many of which are quite expensive. Disability insurance that adequately replaces a person's income is extremely expensive and inaccessible to many people. Some pharmaceutical companies recognize these financial difficulties and provide some free medication to the patient via the physician. However, during difficult economic times, when many individuals cannot afford the cost of medications, the demand greatly exceeds the supply. Not only does illness interfere with income, it also frequently makes it impossible to put any money away for retirement. This can obviously have far-reaching consequences for patients and their families. For many people, there are no good solutions to this problem. However, in many countries, there are government agencies that *will* help, provided that you and your family persist in getting through the red tape. Find a social worker to help you; these people are the experts in the field of social assistance. Lastly, if you have relatives who have the ability to help you financially, don't be embarrassed — ask! The worst that can happen is that they will say no.

Quality of life is, to a large extent, a personal perception. It reflects the way an individual feels about their state of health as well as about various other aspects of life in general. Many people expect to feel good all the time. Those with IBD learn to recognize that this may not be possible. Accepting that there are going to be some down times is an important step in developing the ability to cope successfully with IBD. Patients who can learn self-reliance will be less tied to their doctors, and this will give them self-confidence and higher self-esteem.

Travel Tips

If you have taken the time to learn about your disease and its treatments, and to learn which medications you can start or adjust on your own and when you should use them, you should feel confident about traveling. (See Chapter 12 for more on this.) Remember, many countries have IBD associations, and their members will be only too happy to help you get appropriate care should you need it. Many continental European countries have at least one hospital with English-speaking staff. Join IAMAT (see the Resources section). Because IBD occurs worldwide, there are physicians and surgeons familiar with the condition worldwide.

Many knowledgeable IBD patients are aware that they can deal with most problems on their own. Sometimes all it takes is a telephone call or e-mail to your gastroenterologist back home, for a little advice or to act as a sounding board.

Don't forget your drugs, and take adequate supplies in your carry-on luggage. If you start to experience symptoms, act promptly. People frequently wait to see if a problem will just settle down on its own. Generally, this is not a good idea when you are away from home. Get travel insurance; if your IBD has been troublesome but has been stable for a few months, you should be able to get insurance, though you may have to pay extra. There are companies that specialize in providing travel insurance for people with disabilities.

If you know what's happening when you experience symptoms, it is often reasonable to try to treat yourself (see Chapter 12). If you can afford to go on a trip, you should be able to afford a telephone call to your gastroenterologist for a bit of advice or reassurance. If your doctor corresponds by e-mail, that's sometimes a better choice, especially when you're in a very different time zone. But e-mail is often not a good choice in an urgent situation, so don't wait too long for an e-mail reply — phone. Or, go to a hospital. If you don't know what's happening or you are not sure, *it is foolish to take chances*. In this situation, seek prompt medical assistance. If you feel it would be useful for the local doctor to speak to your gastroenterologist, you can request this and offer to pay for the communication, be it a phone call or a fax.

Employers and IBD

Crohn's disease, and to a lesser extent ulcerative colitis, has always had a bad reputation in the business world. Many employers are reluctant to hire people with IBD, although in practice this discrimination is illegal. The perception is that the IBD patient will be ill frequently and will miss work. In fact, this may never happen. Patients and their doctors have become so good at dealing with most IBD problems on an outpatient basis that many people can keep working when they are ill, with the loss of very few days, if any.

In many ways, IBD patients are ideal employees. Most become toughened by the illness and are more likely to come to work when suffering relatively minor illnesses that would keep many otherwise healthy people at home. IBD patients are conscious of the risk of a flare-up and of having to miss significant periods of work. As a result, they generally try not to miss work for any other reason.

Studies have examined discrimination against people with Crohn's disease in both school and the workplace. In one study, students with Crohn's lost significantly more days of school than healthy students but were as successful academically, as measured by the courses they completed and whether they entered university. Although discrimination against a potential employee on the basis of an illness is illegal, many Crohn's patients feel that they have been rejected for this reason, even though another excuse may have been given. As a result of such experiences, up to 30 percent of Crohn's patients conceal their illness from employers.

Insurance and IBD

For many years, patients and their physicians have known that IBD is used as a reason to refuse insurance or to charge a high premium. Groups in several countries have studied the insurance industry's attitude to people with IBD and also looked at the issue from the patients' point of view. The perception in the insurance industry is that those with IBD may have some difficulty obtaining life insurance.

Patients who are rejected for one type of insurance often neglect to apply for any other type. Representatives of the insurance industry have pointed out that some of the rejections have nothing to do with the diagnosis of IBD and are related to other factors, family history being one example. Unquestionably, disability and premature death due to IBD have decreased significantly in the past 50 years. From doctors' point of view, there is only a minor difference in life expectancy between most sufferers of IBD and the general population. Yet this minor difference is important to the insurance companies, which are, after all, in business.

Strategies for Insurance Applications

Don't be discouraged from applying for insurance just because you have been rejected for one type. And don't give up because you have been rejected by one company; fellow members of your local chapter of the Crohn's and colitis association may be able to guide you to a more empathetic insurance carrier. If you are rejected for one type of insurance (disability, for example), don't give up on all types. You may still be able to get life insurance, mortgage insurance and so on.

If you have Crohn's disease and you've had a flare-up or surgery, it's probably a good idea to wait at least 6 months before applying for insurance. The longer you go without active disease, the greater the likelihood of getting regular insurance with no extra premium.

Since it is somewhat difficult for people with Crohn's disease to acquire benefits, it is important to try to stay at the same job, especially if you are covered in a group insurance plan. Before you do change employment, consider carefully whether your benefits are transferable.

Your doctor will likely be asked to complete a form for your application. It is sometimes very helpful if your doctor adds a letter describing your general health status and your ability to work. This helps the insurance company assess your risk and usually makes your chance of being accepted higher. Your doctor can point out that you are a "good citizen" — you have not lost time from work, you are able to participate in community activities and you have not had much disability — if that is the case.

14

Looking Ahead

Research into causes and treatments of IBD is moving forward on many fronts. The use of genetic engineering in laboratory animals continues to generate excitement because it is possible to create individual immunological defects — known as gene knockout models — allowing researchers to study one particular aspect of a disease or the immune reaction at a time. This will lead to more understanding, and newer and better therapies.

Drug researchers are continuing to search for drugs that act locally in the intestine or hit a specific target in the abnormal immune reaction and then promptly become inactivated, so that side effects are reduced. Nanoparticles are part of an innovative drug administration system that can deliver small molecules of medication directly into inflamed areas. In an effort to reduce costs of some of the newer, expensive biologicals, a new category of drugs, known as biosimilars (also known as subsequent entry biologics [SEBs] in Canada) is being developed. These drugs, which may be thought of as generic versions of biologicals, are currently in clinical trials. As always, chance observations, like the ones regarding nicotine and heparin (see Chapter 6), will be pursued. Future research will also focus on the field of pharmacogenetics, which is the science of using genetic information to predict how well someone will respond to a particular drug or group of drugs. This is the dawn of personalized medicine.

Cancer researchers are using molecular genetics and related technology to look for blood, stool or tissue tests that may replace surveillance colonoscopy. Molecular imaging is a new application in gastrointestinal endoscopy. It is expected that this technology will enhance our ability to detect early colon cancer. Meanwhile, virtual colonoscopy, which surveys the colon with a CT scanner (CT colonography), has come of age. While it cannot provide the tissue samples needed to look for dysplasia, it may prove to be useful in combination with blood or stool tests. So far, the bowel still has to be cleaned out, but virtual colonoscopy is much faster than the endoscopic variety. There are now programs to allow computers to "subtract" the stool in your colon from the surrounding tissues by a process known as fecal tagging. When this technique is market-ready, you won't have to take a prep before the exam. Virtual colonoscopy can also be done with an MR machine (MR colonography), but this is not as well accepted so far. Like CT colonography, you still have to take a prep. The advantage of MR is that it is safe for most people, since there is no radiation.

The role of laparoscopic surgery (using multiple little incisions instead of one big one) in IBD has evolved to the point where it is commonly used, resulting in shorter hospital stays and more rapid recovery for many patients. The use of strictureplasty surgery to preserve bowel has expanded; the procedure has been used recently for some colon strictures, which were always resected in the past. Small bowel transplantation has continued to be a challenge, but efforts in this area continue. When this procedure becomes more successful, it will represent an important step forward for patients with small bowel Crohn's disease who require multiple resections, and for those who are already severely disabled because of a surgically shortened small bowel. Stem cell therapy is in its infancy, with the promise of more new treatments and the prospect of "growing" new pieces of intestine.

There are many thousands of researchers, clinicians and patients all over the world interested in solving the mysteries of IBD. There is every reason to be optimistic that the causes of IBD will be found someday, and we can expect that such discoveries will lead to improved treatments and, ultimately, to cures.

APPENDIX 1

Drugs Commonly Used to Treat IBD

M any drugs are used to treat IBD and its complications; this table focuses on those that relate most specifically to IBD. Note that some are available as generic (no-name) products, and that the list of brand names is not exhaustive.

Drugs Commonly Used to Treat IBD *(as of May 2011)*

Drug Type	Generic Names	Brand Names
Source of 5-ASA	mesalamine/mesalazine (5-aminosalicylate, 5-ASA), prodrugs *(require bacteria to release 5-ASA)* • balsalazide • olsalazine • sulfasalazine	 Colazal* Dipentum Azulfidine,* Salazopyrin†
	mesalamine/mesalazine (5-aminosalicylate, 5-ASA), *delayed or extended-release (acid-resistant coat)*	Apriso,* Asacol, Lialda,* Mesasal,† Mezavant,† Pentasa, Salofalk†
	mesalamine (5-aminosalicylate, 5-ASA), *rectal (liquid enema or suppository)*	Canasa*, Pentasa, Salofalk,† Rowasa,*

Drug Type	Generic Names	Brand Names
Glucocorticoids (commonly known as "steroids"); not the same as anabolic steroids (see Chapter 6)	Prednisone, prednisolone hydrocortisone (rectal, liquid) hydrocortisone (rectal, foam) budesonide (oral) budesonide (rectal) betamethasone (rectal)	Liquid Pred Syrup,* Winpred† Pediapred,† others Cortenema,† Colocort* Cortifoam, Entocort EC† Entocort† Betnesol†
Immunosuppressives	azathioprine 6-mercaptopurine (6-MP) methotrexate cyclosporine tacrolimus mycophenolate mofetil thalidomide lenalidomide	Imuran Purinethol Rheumatrex, others Sandimmune (IV), Neoral (oral) Prograf CellCept Thalomid* Revlimid
Biologicals	infliximab adalimumab certolizumab pegol golimumab ustekinemab natalizumab etanercept filgrastim (G-CSF) sargramostim (GM-CSF)	Remicade Humira Cimzia* Simponi Stelara Tysabri* Enbrel Neupogen Leukine*
Stem cells	Adult human stem cells	Prochymal

Drug Type	Generic Names	Brand Names
Antidiarrheals	loperamide diphenoxylate codeine	Imodium Lomotil
Enteral diet products	—	Ensure plus, Boost plus, others
Bowel cleanout products	polyethylene glycol-electrolyte solution	Colyte, GoLYTELY, Klean-Prep,† NuLyte-ly,* Peglyte,† Bi-Peg-lyte,† Gavi-Lyte-C,* GaviLyte-G,* MoviPrep,* TriLyte,* OCL*
	PEG 3350	Restoralax,† Miral-ax,* Lax-A-Day,† Dulcolax Balance,* others
	picosulfate-magnesium oxide-citric acid	Pico-Salax
Antibiotics	ciprofloxacin metronidazole	Cipro Flagyl
Lactose digestive	lactase	many products available in the United States and Canada
Fiber digestive	Alpha-galactosidase	Beano
Unclassified	lidocaine jelly botulinum toxin A ursodiol (ursodeoxycholic acid)	Xylocaine Botox Actigall,* Urso

* United States only
† Canada only

APPENDIX 2

Lactose-free Diet

For some people with lactose intolerance, symptom control is simply a matter of avoiding milk and obvious milk products, but there are many people who have to be much more vigilant. This table provides you with a lactose-free diet; see Chapter 5 for more information.

Type of food	Foods recommended	Foods to avoid
Milk and milk products	Lactose-free milk (commercially readily available), soy milk.	Lactose-reduced milk, regular milk (skim, 2%, whole, chocolate), goat milk, powdered milk, buttermilk, yogurt (including frozen), all cheeses (except very old aged cheeses), cream (sour, whipping, light, half-and-half), ice cream, ice milk.
Breads and Cereals	Most breads (but read labels), breads from kosher bakeries, most cereals (cooked or dry, but read labels – look for the words "lactose" or "milk"), crackers, bagels, croissants.	Cereals containing milk powder, commercial baked products, most waffles and crepes.

Meats	All plain meats, fish, eggs.	Processed meats, commercially prepared meat products (especially if in a batter or cream sauce).
Fruits and Vegetables	All fruits, vegetables, and their juices, except for those on opposite list, legumes (peas, beans, lentils, chickpeas), nuts, seeds, peanut butter, tofu.	Instant potatoes, processed or commercially prepared potato and vegetable products, commercial fruit-pie fillings.
Soups	Soups made without milk or cream, consommé, broths.	Soups made with milk or cream, commercial soups containing lactose.
Fats and Oils	Butter, lard, milk-free margarine, shortening, oils, mayonnaise.	Margarine containing lactose or milk, cream (if more than 1 tbsp).
Confections	Dark chocolate, various candies (read labels), popsicles	Milk chocolate
Desserts	Soy ice cream, kosher ice cream, plain meringue.	Puddings, sherbet, commercially prepared desserts (cakes, pies, cookies), frozen yogurt.
Beverages	Plain coffee, tea, soft drinks, fruit juices, beer, wine, liquor.	Miscellaneous products (read labels)

APPENDIX 3

Calcium Intake Assessment Guide

Use this guide to estimate your daily calcium intake, using the tables on pages 223–225.

A Guideline to Dietary Sources of Calcium

Including milk or other dairy products in your daily diet makes it fairly easy to meet your daily calcium requirement. However, if dairy product consumption is limited, careful meal planning including other high calcium foods is necessary. You might need a calcium supplement, but first check with your physician or dietitian/nutritionist. *Too much calcium can be as harmful for you as too little calcium.* Aim for 800 to 1,200 milligrams of calcium per day (men and premenopausal women). The target for postmenopausal women is somewhat controversial; 1,200 to 1,600 milligrams per day is a reasonable estimate.

If You Are Lactose Intolerant

For patients with severe lactose intolerance, lactose-free milk may be the best and easiest way to meet your calcium requirement, particularly if cheese is not consumed on a daily basis. Making milk lactose-free doesn't alter the calcium content.

What's a "Serving"?

What does a serving look like? Use your hand to estimate cups (milliliters), ounces (grams) and portions. Let your fist, thumb and palm be your portion guide. (Amounts cited refer to a woman's hand of average size.) A thumb = 1 ounce (30 g) of cheese; a palm = 3 ounces (90 g); a handful = 1 or 2 ounces (30 to 60 g); thumb tip = 1 teaspoon (5 ml); and a fist = 1 cup (250 ml).

Calcium Intake Record

Use the portion sizes noted above to help you. **Do not record anything consumed less than once a week.** If you take any calcium tablets, list them below, and *remember to add to your total:*

a. name of product:

b. amount of calcium per tablet:

c. number of tablets taken per day:

Note: Items not listed below may contain calcium, but most will have less than 50 grams per serving. Some food items listed can have a varying amount of calcium depending on preparation method and production source.

Some foods, such as beet greens, spinach and rhubarb, contain calcium as cited below, but they also contain oxalic acid, which interferes with calcium absorption, so that the amount of calcium available for absorption is less than listed. You can get more information about this on the Internet.

Also, the calcium content has been rounded off for convenience. Mixed dishes (e.g., lasagna, pizza, wieners and beans) are not included, as amounts will vary depending on milk-product content.

Intake Record

Group 1
each choice contains
300 milligrams calcium

	Portion	Amount per day	Number of days per week	Total intake
Skim milk	1 cup (250 ml)			
2% milk	1 cup (250 ml)			
Whole milk	1 cup (250 ml)			
Buttermilk	1 cup (250 ml)			
Yogurt	1 cup (250 ml)			
Gruyere cheese	1 oz (30 g)			
Parmesan cheese	1 oz (30 g)			
Smelt, canned, with bones*	4 or 5 medium			

Group 2
each choice contains
200 milligrams calcium

	Portion	Amount per day	Number of days per week	Total intake
Brick cheese	1 oz (30 g)			
Cheddar cheese	1 oz (30 g)			
Cottage cheese, creamed	1 cup (250 ml)			
Edam cheese	1 oz (30 g)			
Liederkranz cheese	1 oz (30 g)			
Process cheese	1 oz (30 g)			
Roquefort cheese	1 oz (30 g)			
Swiss cheese	1 oz (30 g)			
Salmon, canned, with bones*	3 1/2 oz (100g)			
Sardines, with bones*	5 medium (2 oz/60 g)			
Rhubarb, cooked	1/2 cup (125 ml)			

*Bones of canned smelt, salmon and sardines
 must be eaten if calcium content is to be counted.*

Group 3
each choice contains
100 milligrams calcium

	Portion	Amount per day	Number of days per week	Total intake
Blue cheese	1 oz (30 g)			
Cottage cheese, uncreamed,	1–2% fat 2/3 cup (150 ml)			
Limburger cheese	1 oz (30 g)			
Ice cream	1/2 cup (125 ml)			
Ice milk	1/2 cup (125 ml)			
Tofu	2.5 × 1 inch (6 × 2 cm) block or approx. 3 oz (90 g)			
Custard, baked or boiled	1/2 cup (125 ml)			
Cream soups	3/4 cup (200 ml)			
Cream of Wheat, instant, cooked	1/2 cup (125 ml)			
Oatmeal, instant, cooked	1/2 cup (125 ml)			
Beet greens, cooked	1/2 cup (125 ml)			
Broccoli, cooked	2/3 cup (150 ml)			
Collards, cooked	1/2 cup (125 ml)			
Dandelion greens, cooked	1/2 cup (125 ml)			
Kale, cooked	3/4 cup (200 ml)			
Okra, cooked	8 to 9 pods (3 1/2 oz/100 g)			
Mustard greens, cooked	1/2 cup (125 ml)			
Spinach, cooked	2/3 cup (150 ml)			
Turnip greens, cooked	1/2 cup (125 ml)			
Figs, dried	5 medium			
Oysters	4 medium			
Blackstrap molasses	1 tbsp (15 ml)			

Group 4 *each choice contains 50 milligrams calcium*	Portion	Amount per day	Number of days per week	Total intake
Coffee cream	2 oz (60 ml)			
Half-and-half	2 oz (60 ml)			
Sour cream	2 oz (60 ml)			
Soy milk	1 cup (250 ml)			
Whipping cream	2 oz (60 ml)			
Milk chocolate	1 oz (30 g)			
Cabbage, cooked	3/4 cup (200 ml)			
Green beans, cooked	1 cup (250 ml)			
Orange, fresh	1 medium			
Almonds, roasted	12 to 15			
Brazil nuts	8 to 9			
Mussels	1, or 3/4 oz (20 g)			
Scallops	1, or 3/4 oz (20 g)			
Shrimp, canned	1/2 cup (125 ml/3 1/2 oz/100 g)			
Grand Total				
Average Daily Total				

APPENDIX 4

Fructose and Sorbitol Content of Fruit and Fruit Juices

Fruit or Fruit Juice	Fructose (grams per 1/2 cup/ 125 ml)	Sorbitol (grams per 1/2 cup/ 125 ml)
Apple	6.0	0.5
Blackberry	3.4	0.0
Cherry, sweet	7.0	1.4
Grape	6.5	trace
Orange	2.4	0.0
Peach	1.1	0.9
Pear	6.6	2.1
Pineapple	1.4	0.0
Prune	14.0	12.7
Raspberry	2.0	0.0
Strawberry	2.2	0.0

APPENDIX 5

High-Iron Foods

Food	Serving size	Iron (mg)
Meat and Alternates		
Pork liver, cooked	3 oz (90 g)	26.1
Beef kidney, cooked	3 oz (90 g)	11.8
Beef or chicken liver, cooked	3 oz (90 g)	8.0
Baked beans with pork in tomato sauce	1 cup (250 ml)	4.9
Chili with beans	1 cup (250 ml)	4.5
Corned beef	3 oz (90 g)	3.9
Liverwurst	2 oz (60 g)	3.2
Seeds: pumpkin, sesame	1/4 cup (50 ml)	3.2
Beef, pork, veal, ham, roasted	3 oz (90 g)	3.0
Fruits and Vegetables		
Prune juice	1/2 cup (125 ml)	5.5
Spinach, cooked	1/2 cup (125 ml)	3.4
Cereals		
Whole grain and dry enriched	3/4 cup (2 ml)	4.5

APPENDIX 6

Controlled-Oxalate Diet

This diet is used to reduce kidney stone risk for people prone to calcium oxalate stones. The following foods are high in oxalates (containing more than 10 milligrams per average serving) and should be avoided completely. Those marked with an asterisk (*) have a very high oxalate content.

Beverages: draft beer, stout, Ovaltine, tea, cocoa
Limit coffee to 1 cup (250 ml) per day.

Vegetables: beans (green, wax, dried), beets (tops, roots, greens), celery, collard greens, dandelion greens, eggplant, leeks, okra, parsley, plantain, spinach,* summer squash, sweet potato

Fruits: blackberries, Concord grapes, currants (red and black), figs, gooseberries, plums, prunes, raspberries, rhubarb,* strawberries, tangerines and peels from grapefruit, lemon, lime, and orange

Breads and grains: grits, lentils, soybean crackers, soybeans, wheat germ, whole wheat bread (more than two slices of daily)

Miscellaneous: chocolate, cocoa, nuts (cashews, almonds, pecans), peanut butter, tofu

These restrictions should be combined with an intake of at least 8 cups (2 liters) of fluid daily, plus some lemon juice, which contains potassium citrate, to inhibit stone formation.

APPENDIX 7

Simple Strengthening Exercises

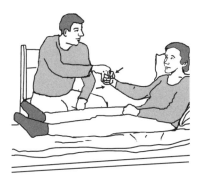

Figure 1 – squeeze fingers

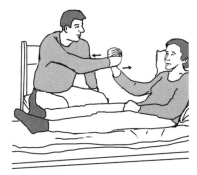

Figure 2 – pull hands

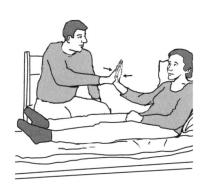

Figure 3 – push hands

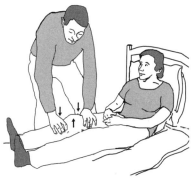

Figure 4 – bend knee

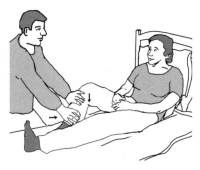

Figure 5 – straighten knee

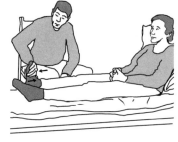

Figure 6 – pull foot

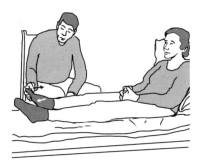

Figure 7 – push foot

In figures 2–7, the helper is providing resistance to the patient's actions.

Glossary

Abdominoperineal resection: an operation to remove the rectum and anus; it requires incisions in both the abdomen and the perineum.

Abscess: a localized collection of pus (living and dead white blood cells and a mixture of live and dead bacteria).

Acute: of rapid onset and short duration.

Adenocarcinoma: any cancer originating in glandular tissues such as those found in the gastrointestinal tract. These usually begin as adenomas (see Chapter 10).

Adenoma: a new growth of glandular tissue; in the gastrointestinal tract, usually seen as a polyp.

Adhesions: bands of scar tissue that are usually a result of surgery and connect the area of surgery to another structure such as a section of intestine or the peritoneum.

Anal canal: the channel connecting the rectum to the outside world.

Anal sphincter: a ring of muscle surrounding the anal canal, controlling the opening and closing of the anus.

Anastomosis: a surgically created connection of separate or severed tubular hollow organs.

Anemia: abnormally low level of red blood cells or hemoglobin in the blood.

Anus: the lower opening of the anal canal.

Appliance: the plastic bag used to collect stool coming out of an ileostomy or colostomy.

ASA: the drug acetylsalicylic acid.

Ascending colon: section of colon running from the ileocecal valve to the hepatic flexure.

Barium enema: an X-ray examination of the colon, and sometimes the end of the ileum, using a suspension of barium sulfate, which appears white on X-ray film.

Barium small bowel enema: an X-ray examination of the small intestine in which a radiologist injects a suspension of barium sulfate through a small plastic tube that has been inserted into the intestine through the nose.

Biliary: pertaining to bile, a fluid that delivers bile salts to the small intestine to help digestion of fat, and carries some toxins and waste from the liver into the bowel; the bile ducts ("bil-iary tree") extend from inside the liver to the duodenum.

Biologicals: also known as biologics; a new class of drugs that target specific molecules in the inflammatory process.

Biopsy: a tissue sample removed for examination under a microscope. An entire area of tissue may be removed or only a little bit. Although biopsies are often taken to look for cancer, many other tissue abnormalities are also diagnosed through biopsy.

Brooke ileostomy: most commonly used form of ileostomy, invented by British surgeon Bryan Brooke; *see also* Ileostomy.

Capsule endoscopy (The PillCam®): a method for examining the small intestine. A tiny camera in a capsule is swallowed, and images are later downloaded onto a computer. The technology is being refined to also permit colon examination.

CAT scan: *see* CT scan.

Cecum: a large, blind pouch, forming the beginning of the colon on the lower right side of the abdomen, where the appendix is.

Chronic: lasting for a long time or frequently recurring.

Colectomy: surgical removal of part or all of the colon; often specified as total (including the rectum; also called "proctocolectomy"), or subtotal (excluding the rectum).

Colitis: inflammation of the colon.

Colon: the large intestine (or large bowel), extending from the cecum to the rectum, though the rectum is often referred to separately.

Colonoscopy: an examination of the colon with a flexible instrument inserted into the rectum.

Commensal: a microbe that normally lives in close contact with a human or animal without causing any harm. From the time we are born, we all have commensals in our gastro-intestinal systems.

Constipation: bowel movements that are harder or less frequent than normal; may also refer to passage of an inadequate volume of stool.

CT colonography: a CT examination of the

colon in which a small amount of liquid contrast medium and some air are inserted into the colon through a small tube placed in the rectum; the test takes just a few minutes and the result is a video image of the colon, focused on the inner lining.

CT enteroclysis: a CT examination of the small intestine in which a radiologist injects a liquid contrast medium through a small plastic tube that has been inserted into the intestine through the nose.

CT enterography: a CT examination of the small intestine in which the patient drinks a liquid contrast medium.

CT scan: computerized axial tomography, which takes X-rays of "slices" of the body; also known as CAT scan.

Cytokines: chemicals released by immune cells and responsible for coordinating an immune response.

Descending colon: part of the colon running down the left side, from the splenic flexure to the sigmoid colon.

Diarrhea: bowel movements that are softer, looser or more frequent than normal.

Duodenum: the first part of the small intestine, starting at the lower end of the stomach and extending to the jejunum.

Elemental diet: a sterilized manufactured diet including protein (as amino acids) and carbohydrate (as glucose) and vitamins, minerals and a small amount of fat. This diet requires little or no digestion. *See also* Polymeric diet.

Endoscope: an instrument used to examine the inside of a part of the body.

Enteral diet: Strictly speaking, any diet taken by mouth, as opposed to a parenteral diet, which is administered intravenously. But the term is applied to a sterilized, manufactured, liquid diet that may be drunk or administered through a tube into the stomach or intestine.

Enteritis: inflammation of the small intestine.

Enteroscopy: examination of the small intestine with an endoscope.

Enterostomal therapist: a nurse who specializes in the care of ostomies and some of their complications; also known as an ET.

Enzymes: proteins or conjugated proteins, produced by living organisms, which speed chemical reactions such as the digestion (breakdown) of other substances.

Esophagogastroduodenoscopy: examination of the esophagus, stomach and duodenum with an endoscope; also known as EGD or OGD.

Esophagus: the swallowing tube, a muscular tube-like structure that propels food from the throat into the stomach.

Expert patients: patients who are extremely knowledgeable about their condition, and its management.

False urge: a strong but mistaken feeling that a bowel movement is going to occur; a symptom of rectal inflammation.

Feces: *see* Stool.

Fissure: a break in surface tissue, such as skin or mucosa; may be superficial, as in an anal fissure (a tear in the skin of the anal canal), or a deep crack-like ulcer extending into the wall of the GI tract, as in Crohn's disease.

Fistula: an abnormal connection between two hollow structures (e.g., two segments of intestine, or a segment of intestine and the bladder), or between a hollow structure and the skin surface.

5-ASA: the drug 5-aminosalicylate.

Flare: an increase in activity of a disease.

Flexible sigmoidoscopy: examination of the rectum and sigmoid colon with an endoscope; may include some or all of the descending colon, and some of the transverse colon.

Gastroenterologist: a medical specialist in the diagnosis and treatment of diseases of the stomach, intestines and associated organs (gastrointestinal tract).

Gastrointestinal tract: the mouth, esophagus, stomach, small intestine, large intestine (colon), rectum, anus, liver, biliary system and pancreas.

GI tract: gastrointestinal tract.

Glucocorticoids: a family of steroid hormones, both synthetic and naturally occurring, that have anti-inflammatory properties.

Growth failure: an effect that any chronic disease may have on a child who has not finished growing. Growth is usually slowed but may stop completely; reduced activity of the disease, especially in combination with improved nutrition, usually corrects the problem.

Hepatic flexure: a sharp bend in the colon just below the liver, where the ascending colon becomes the transverse colon.

IBD: inflammatory bowel disease, which includes Crohn's disease and ulcerative colitis; some people also include microscopic colitis, SCAD (*see below*) and Behçet's disease.

Ileitis: any inflammation of the ileum; the term is often used as a synonym for Crohn's disease of the ileum.

Ileocecal valve: short area of muscle thickening located where the ileum joins the colon, which controls the release of the fluid contents of the ileum into the colon.

Ileostomy: surgically created opening from the ileum to the abdominal surface, to allow stool to pass from the body into a plastic bag.

Ileum: last portion of the small intestine, extending from the jejunum to the cecum.

Immunomodulator: a drug that modifies immune function.

Immunosuppressives: a group of medications whose common characteristic is that they reduce activity of part of the immune system. They represent one group of immunomodulators.

Inflammation: a localized protective reaction to injury or infection, characterized by pain, swelling, redness, heat and sometimes loss of function.

Irritable bowel syndrome (IBS): a disorder of the GI tract usually involving an abnormal bowel habit and abdominal discomfort. IBS can mimic some features of Crohn's disease but does not usually cause weight loss. It does not cause bowel inflammation.

Jejunum: upper portion of the small intestine, connecting the duodenum to the ileum.

Kock ileostomy: an ileostomy that allows stool to be collected in an internal reservoir, called a Kock pouch, instead of an external bag; also known as a "continent ileostomy."

Kock pouch: a reservoir for stool, surgically constructed from the ileum.

Lactase: an enzyme in the mucosa (inner lining) of the small intestine that breaks down lactose into two simpler sugars, glucose and galactose.

Lactose: a sugar in dairy products, also found in some processed foods and medications.

Lactose intolerance: a partial or complete inability to digest lactose, generally resulting in abdominal pain, excess lower bowel gas and sometimes diarrhea; also known as "lactase deficiency."

Laparoscopic surgery: often called "keyhole surgery"; instead of one large incision, the surgeon uses several very small incisions, and operates by using a video system. Benefits can include less pain after surgery, less time in the hospital, more rapid recovery and much smaller scars than would result from conventional surgery.

Lesion: a localized pathological change or injury to body tissue; a cancer is a lesion, and so is a scratch.

Leukocyte scan: a test using radioactively labeled white blood cells (leukocytes) to locate areas of inflammation.

Liquid-diet therapy: a treatment for Crohn's disease using a diet consisting entirely of sterilized liquids, mostly manufactured high-energy products; sometimes used as a nutritional source for people with ulcerative colitis, but it is not a treatment on its own.

Lymphoma: cancer arising in lymphoid tissue, which is present in many locations throughout the body, mainly as lymph glands, and is part of the immune system.

Mesentery: a fan-shaped piece of tissue that acts like a sling, holding the small intestine. Within this sling are lymph glands, fat and blood vessels.

Microbes: Tiny living organisms, mostly visible only with a microscope. Some microbes cause diseases, whereas others are essential for a healthy life. The three main types of microbes are bacteria, viruses, and fungi, which includes yeasts.

Microbiota: The microbial population in an individual.

Modular product: a manufactured nutritional product that supplies a single nutrient.

MR: magnetic resonance imaging, a computerized imaging technique; also known as MRI.

MR colonography: an MR examination of the colon in which water is inserted into the colon through a small tube placed in the rectum.

MR enterography: an MR examination of the small intestine.

Mucosa: the inner lining of any hollow structure in the body.

Mucous fistula: a surgically created connection between part of the GI tract and the skin; it differs from an ostomy in that the portion of intestine leading to the mucous fistula is disconnected from the flow of bowel contents.

Mucus: nature's lubricant, normally produced by glands of the mucosa.

Osmosis: diffusion of a fluid across a membrane.

Ostomy: surgically created connection between two portions of the GI tract, or between a portion carrying bowel contents and the skin.

Parenteral: entering the body by a route other than the GI tract, such as by intravenous or intramuscular injection.

Parenteral nutrition: a technique of supplying nutrition directly into the bloodstream, bypassing the intestine.

Patient passport: a written or electronic summary of the essential details of a person's disease.

Pelvic pouch: a reservoir surgically constructed from the ileum, as a substitute for the rectum.

Perforation: a hole right through the wall of a hollow structure.

Perianal: around the anus, but the term is also used to refer to the area within the anal canal.

Perineum: the area between the anus and the posterior boundary of the genitals.

Peritoneum: a thin, tough membrane lining the abdominal cavity and folding inward to enclose some of the abdominal organs.

Peritonitis: inflammation of the peritoneum.

PET scan: a relatively new form of medical imaging, using the metabolic activity of tissues to produce a three-dimensional image or picture of selected areas of the body.

Phlegmon: an infected, inflamed mass of tissue.

Phytochemicals: health-promoting chemicals found in plants.

PN: *see* Parenteral nutrition.

Polymeric diet: a synthetic diet that contains food components in forms requiring at least some digestion; *see also* Elemental diet.

Pouchitis: inflammation of either a Kock pouch or a pelvic pouch.

Probiotics: living microbes, believed to be health-promoting.

Proctocolectomy: *see* Colectomy.

Rectum: the last part of the colon, from the sigmoid colon to the anal canal.

Resection: surgical removal of an organ or part of an organ.

Sacroiliitis: inflammation of the sacroiliac joints, at the back of the pelvis.

SCAD: Segmental colitis associated with diverticulitis.

Serosa: the outer lining of the GI tract, present everywhere except in the esophagus and the lower half of the rectum.

Seton: a loop of thread, wire or gauze used temporarily to keep a fistula open.

Short bowel syndrome: a condition of chronic diarrhea and reduced absorption of food, due to surgical removal or bypass of a major portion of the small intestine.

Sigmoid colon: part of the colon connecting the descending colon to the rectum.

Sigmoidoscopy: examination of the rectum and sigmoid colon with an endoscope; *see also* Flexible sigmoidoscopy.

Sign: a finding made during the course of a physical examination, such as an enlarged liver.

Small bowel series: an X-ray examination of the small intestine in which the patient drinks a suspension of barium sulfate.

Sphincter: a ring of muscle that opens and closes, to control the passage of something.

Splenic flexure: part of the colon just below the spleen, where the transverse colon turns abruptly to become the descending colon.

Steroids: commonly refers to a large number of hormones with a similar chemical structure. They include glucocorticoid steroids (which reduce inflammation), male sex hormones (such as the so-called anabolic steroids sometimes misused by athletes), female sex hormones and others.

Stoma: the surgically constructed opening of an ostomy.

Stool: a collective term for the various components discharged at the end of the GI tract. Whether this material comes out of the rectum, a colostomy or an ileostomy, as a liquid or a solid, it is still called stool.

Stricture: an abnormal area of narrowing of a hollow organ or structure.

Strictureplasty: a surgical technique that widens an area of narrowing, instead of removing it; also known as "stricturoplasty."

Suppository: rapidly dissolving form of solid medication that is inserted through the anus into the rectum.

Symptom: something abnormal perceived by the patient, such as fatigue or pain.

Tenesmus: an intense urge to have a bowel movement, relieved partially or not at all by the passage of material from the rectum, whether it is stool, blood or gas; frequently associated with an inability to pass anything. Tenesmus is a symptom of rectal inflammation.

TNF: stands for tumor necrosis factor; the best-known drugs in the biologicals group block the action of TNF, a cytokine that is overactive in many cases of IBD.

Topical: medication applied directly to the area affected; when being used to treat inflammation in the anal area or rectum, a suppository is an example.

Toxic megacolon: the most serious complication of an attack of acute colitis. Some or all of the colon becomes paralyzed and swells up with gas, stretching the wall.

TPN: total parenteral nutrition; *see* Parenteral.

Trace elements: elements required by the body in very tiny amounts, such as zinc and chromium.

Transverse colon: part of the colon running across the upper abdomen, from the hepatic flexure to the splenic flexure.

Ulcer: a break in a lining; an open sore on an arm *is* a skin ulcer, for example. The ulcers of the small bowel or colon that occur in ulcerative colitis or Crohn's disease have nothing to do with duodenal or stomach ulcers.

Ulcerative proctitis: ulcerative colitis that only involves the rectum.

Ultrasound: a technique for examining tissues using sound waves.

Upper GI series: X-ray examination of the esophagus, stomach and duodenum; the patient drinks a suspension of barium sulfate, and several X-rays are taken.

Resources

Organizations

In addition to the many helpful books and websites available on Crohn's disease and ulcerative colitis, there are chapters of the Crohn's and Colitis Foundation and the United Ostomy Association across the United States and Canada, and Crohn's and colitis associations around the world; check the Internet or your telephone book for your local chapter.

United States

Crohn's & Colitis Foundation of America
386 Park Avenue South
17th Floor
New York, NY 10016
Phone: 800-932-2423
E-mail: info@www.ccfa.org
URL: http://www.ccfa.org

United Ostomy Associations of America
UOAA
P.O. Box 512
Northfield MN 55057-0512
Phone: 800-826-0826
E-mail: info@ostomy.org
URL: http://www.ostomy.org

Canada

Crohn's and Colitis Foundation of Canada
600-60 St. Clair Avenue East
Toronto, ON M4T 1N5
Phone: 416-920-5035
Toll-free: 1-800-387-1479
E-mail: ccfc@ccfc.ca
URL: http://www.ccfc.ca

United Ostomy Association of Canada Inc.
344 Bloor St. West, Suite 501
Toronto, ON M5S 3A7
Phone: 416-595-5452
Toll-free: 1-888-969-9698
E-mail: info1@ostomycanada.ca
URL: http://www.ostomycanada.ca

United Kingdom

Crohn's and Colitis UK (formerly NACC)
4 Beaumont House, Sutton Road
St Albans, Herts AL1 5HH
Phone: 0845-130-2233
E-mail: info@CrohnsAndColitis.org.uk
URL: http://www.nacc.org.uk

Europe

European Federation of Crohn's & Ulcerative Colitis Associations
Rue Vieux Marché aux Grain, 48
Brussels 1000 Belgium
Phone: +32 2 540 84 34
E-Mail: info@efcca.org
URL: http://efcca.org

Australia

Crohn's & Colitis Australia
Level 1, 462 Burwood Road
Hawthorn Victoria 3122
Phone: 61-3-9815-1266
Toll-free: 1-800-138-029
E-mail: info@crohnsandcolitis.com.au
URL: http://www.crohnsandcolitis.com.au

International Association for Medical Assistance to Travellers (IAMAT)

http://www.iamat.org/index.cfm

IAMAT Canada
67 Mowat Avenue, Suite 036
Toronto, ON M6K 3E3
Tel: 416-652-0137 and

2162 Gordon Street
Guelph, ON N1L 1G6
Tel: 519-836-0102
Fax: 519-836-3412

IAMAT USA
1623 Military Road #279
Niagara Falls, NY 14304-1745
Tel: 716-754-4883

IAMAT New Zealand
206 Papanui Road
Christchurch 5

Index

Page numbers in italic indicate a figure, table, or boxed text. For brand names of drugs, see table on pages 216-220.